BASIC & ADVANCE
CARDIAC LIFE SUPPORT

MEDICAL SCHOOL CRASH COURSE

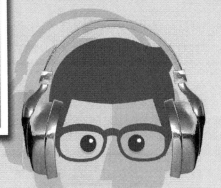

HIGH-YIELD CONTENT REVIEW
Q&A AND "KEY TAKEAWAYS"
TOP 100 TEST QUESTIONS

FOLLOW-ALONG PDF MANUAL

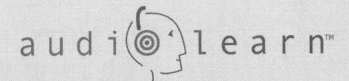

audio learn™

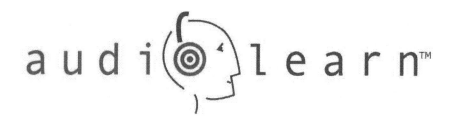

Basic & Advance Cardiac Life Support

Medical School Crash Course™

www.AudioLearn.com

Table of Contents

Preface

The intention of this course is to offer a broad base of information to the potential healthcare provider regarding the basics of Basic Life Support, Advanced Cardiac Life Support, and Advanced Trauma Life Support. Nearly every healthcare provider will face having to care for the critically-ill or critically-injured patient and will need to know how best to stabilize these types of patients so they can receive definitive care.

The first chapter will be an intensive discussion of the assessment of the unconscious patient. These patients represent a unique challenge to the healthcare provider as they cannot verbally relay any symptoms and most are seriously ill, requiring urgent evaluation and management.

In chapter two, there will be a thorough discussion of Basic Life Support for Adults. While Basic Life Support is intended to be used by anyone, there are unique aspects to the provision of this type of vital patient care that are different when a skilled healthcare provider delivers the service as opposed to a lay person.

The third chapter of the course will be a discussion of the Basic Life Support protocols for infants and children. Infants and children have cardiac arrests for different reasons than in adults but still require CPR during an arrest situation. The protocols to be followed by the lay person and healthcare provider alike will be included in this chapter.

In chapter four, the focus of the discussion will be on how the automated external defibrillator works and how it is best put into use in the field. The student will learn how the AED has the potential to save many lives because it quickly restores the rhythm of an adult or child with a non-survivable rhythm strip.

Chapter five of the course is intended to be an introduction into the rhythms seen in Advanced Cardiac Life Support. Each rhythm has unique features that can be identified by the healthcare provider, setting the pace for intervention by the ACLS team.

The algorithms used in the adult patient with an abnormal rhythm or who is in a cardiac arrest situation will be the main topic of discussion in the sixth chapter of the course. Each rhythm and clinical situation has a specific algorithm to follow. The intricacies of these algorithms as they apply to different arrest situations will be covered in that chapter as they apply to the patient with an arrhythmia or who has suffered a cardiorespiratory arrest.

The seventh chapter of the course will be a discussion of the medications used in cardiac arrest situations and in treating arrhythmias. The purposes and dosages of the medications will be covered as part of understanding how they are put into use in various arrhythmia and arrest situations.

The eighth chapter of the course is intended to be an introduction to the basics of pediatric advanced life support or PALS. Children have different common rhythm disturbances and suffer from arrests for very different reasons than adults and require a different approach than is seen in adults who have an arrest situation.

In the ninth chapter of the course, prehospital trauma assessment and management will be discussed. The prehospital rescuer is in a special situation of being able to have a positive impact on the survival of the critically-injured patient and there are protocols for managing these patients that will be the focus of this chapter.

The tenth chapter of the course will include a thorough discussion of Advanced Trauma Life Support or ATLS for adults. Trauma patients can have a variety of injuries and often require intense resuscitation soon after being injured if they are to survive.

The eleventh chapter of the course involves information related to the trauma situations seen in pediatric patients. Pediatric patients are highly likely to be multiply traumatized in an accident or fall and usually require evaluation and treatment of more than one body area after they become injured.

Chapter 1: Initial Assessment of the Unconscious Patient

In many cases, the management of a very sick patient starts with coming upon a patient who is unconscious for a variety of reasons or with observing someone who suddenly or gradually becomes unconscious. This represents a unique medical situation in which there is a seriously ill patient who cannot give you an adequate history. The initial assessment and management of the unconscious patient is the focus of this initial chapter on basic and advanced life support.

Understanding Unconsciousness

The basic finding in unconsciousness is the inability to respond to one's surroundings. Another term for unconsciousness is being in a "coma" or being "comatose", although the implications with these terms is that the person has been in the state for more than just a brief period of time. A person can suddenly become unconscious; however, more likely, they begin with an altered mental status, which affects the way they interact with the environment. Terms used to define an altered mental status is disorientation, confusion, or stupor—all terms that can be used somewhat interchangeably to represent an altered mental status of any kind.

Alterations in mental status may resolve themselves or may progress to full unconsciousness. What this means is that things, such as confusion, stupor, and disorientation are just symptoms along a spectrum from full consciousness to unconsciousness, with all of the above considered a medical emergency that need to be urgently addressed.

The major causes of unconsciousness can be divided into an injury or an illness significant enough to impair the function of the central nervous system (CNS). Drug and alcohol use/abuse can be causes of unconsciousness if the levels are high enough. Choking can cause hypoxia to the brain, resulting in unconsciousness. Low blood sugar can starve the brain of nutrients necessary to function, leading to unconsciousness. Dehydration can cause low blood pressure, low perfusion to the brain, and subsequent unconsciousness (which might be brief and related only to standing up). Cardiac arrhythmias can render a person unconscious by virtue of not perfusing the brain. Blood loss can cause hypoperfusion to the brain and subsequent CNS dysfunction.

During a period of unconsciousness, the major symptom noted is the inability to be responsive to the environment. In general, in includes the inability to respond to visual, auditory, touch, or pain sensation, although patients may still retain the ability to respond to pain and would still be judged as being unconscious if they met the other criteria.

Following an episode of unconsciousness, the individual will likely have amnesia for events occurring during the unconscious event and may have amnesia of events leading to the episode or events following the episode. Post-coma confusion is common a is drowsiness and headache. Patients may remain lightheaded after they come back to consciousness and may have, throughout the events leading up to the unconsciousness or afterward, loss of bowel or bladder control.

Other symptoms that may be present shortly after restoration of consciousness include stroke-like symptoms (such as hemiparesis and aphasia), shortness of breath, ongoing confusion, overall weakness, palpitations, weak cough reflex, and cyanosis. Patients who are unconscious are not simply sleeping and usually have significant CNS dysfunction affecting the brain in a global way. They will not respond to shaking and loud sounds.

First Aid Approaches to Altered Mental Status

The first part of the assessment involves a brief visualization of the patient. Are they breathing? Do they have a pulse? The absence of either of these two things places the situation beyond simply being unconscious. This falls under the category of cardiorespiratory arrest and needs urgent intervention as failing to intervene within a couple of minutes means certain brain damage and likely death.

If the patient has not yet reached full unconsciousness, an assessment begins by asking some basic questions. Ask the patient their name, the date, the day of the week, and where they think they are. Sometimes it takes several questions along these lines in order to fully assess the patient's mental status. Patients with an altered mental status may know their name and birthdate but will be completely confused as to their location and the time. These latter things tend to be deficits first before being able to give personal information about themselves.

If it is determined that the level of consciousness has reached a state where they are unresponsive to their surroundings, 911 should be notified as soon as possible, particularly if there are no resources at the site to adequately treat the patient's cardiopulmonary status.

Airway, breathing, and pulse should be assessed before anything else in the unconscious patient as these things being absent or dysfunctional can quickly kill the person. Any other evaluation should be secondary to those three things.

If the individual is not suspected of having a spinal injury (is not a trauma patient), they need to be rolled to one side with the hip and knee sitting on top bent at a ninety-degree angle. Their airway should be opened by tilting back the head. The goal of putting them on their side is to prevent aspiration of vomitus should the patient unconsciously vomit. A side-lying position is the best way to protect the airway.

Continually monitor the pulse and respiratory status while observing them on their side. The state of unconsciousness is highly unstable and the individual may lose the ability to breathe on their own or may develop a cardiac arrest, changing the approach from one of observation to one of doing cardiopulmonary resuscitation (CPR). All CPR should be done while the person is on their back so they need to be placed on their back again if they meet the criteria for needing CPR.

If, on the other hand, the patient is a known trauma victim and is suspected of having a cervical spine injury, no movement of the body is recommended and the person should remain in the position they are in at the time they are found—only as long as they are able to breathe spontaneously in the position. A jaw-thrust maneuver should replace tilting back the head to open the airway. Sometimes, a jaw-thrust maneuver can make a big difference in the respiratory status of a patient with an impaired respiratory drive or an impairment in their ability to maintain their own airway.

If the unconscious individual is suspected of having a cervical spine injury suddenly vomits, they need to be placed on their side in order to prevent aspiration, which has the potential to compromise the airway. The difference between rolling a trauma patient and a non-trauma patient is that, with a trauma patient, the head and neck must remain in the same position relative to one another throughout the roll as any shifting may compromise the cervical spine.

Special situations exist when the patient has a witnessed loss of consciousness. The first goal is to prevent them from being injured in a fall caused by becoming unconscious. The second goal is to determine if the patient has simply fainted (and will rapidly regain consciousness when lying supine) or has suffered a cardiorespiratory arrest. If they have simply fainted, placing them supine and raising the feet up by about a foot will increase cerebral perfusion.

Another special situation exists when the patient has a loss of consciousness or altered mental status and is a known type 1 or insulin-dependent diabetic. By far and away, the biggest cause of a loss of consciousness or altered mentation in a diabetic is hypoglycemia. Never attempt to give oral sugar solutions, tablets, or anything else orally unless the patient is conscious. If they are conscious, it is appropriate to give them something sweet even if you don't have a blood glucose determination at the time.

A third special circumstance exists if the patient becomes unconscious shortly after choking on something. This might be a typical scenario in a restaurant or dining room. The recommendation for this is to start CPR immediately as chest compressions may dislodge the foreign body. If this fails to improve the patient's status within a minute, look for a loose and visible foreign object. If it is not obviously loose, attempts at dislodging it may push the object further down the airway.

The only choice after this is to continue CPR until emergency medical services (EMS) arrives to manage the patient. The patient should be evaluated every minute or so to see if they are breathing spontaneously or to see if they have effectively dislodged the object.

Things that are definitely contraindicated in managing the unconscious patient is giving them anything to eat or drink, leaving them without constant supervision, placing a pillow under their head (this closes off the airway), or attempting to revive them by splashing them with cold water or hitting them across the face.

Indications for calling 911 immediately include the following:

- The patient is unconscious and is older than 50 years of age.
- The patient is unconscious and is pregnant (at any gestational age).

- The patient is unconscious and has no spontaneous respirations.
- The patient has lost control of his or her bowels or bladder while unconscious.
- The patient is having a seizure (particularly if you do not know if they have a known seizure disorder.
- The patient is a diabetic (even if you haven't documented hypoglycemia).
- The patient has suffered some type of known or suspected trauma.
- The patient has been unconscious for longer than a minute.

Even if the patient has regained consciousness fairly quickly, 911 should be contacted if the patient has an irregular heartbeat, chest pressure/pain, or has any type of focal neurological deficit (such as aphasia or paralysis).

Using the Glasgow Coma Scale (GCS)

In actuality, most patients are not fully conscious or fully awake but is somewhere in between the two. The Glasgow Coma Scale (GCS) can easily provide an objective and reliable measurement of the individual's level of consciousness. It can be done repeatedly and as often as necessary to judge the patient's neurological status.

The revised GCS includes a point range between three and fifteen, where three indicates a deep level of unconsciousness and fifteen represents total alertness. It was first developed to gauge the level of consciousness following a head injury but has expanded to include the assessment of anyone who has an altered level of consciousness for any reason. It is a widely used by first responders, EMS crewmembers, and emergency medicine personnel to indicate to each other the person's level of consciousness. It is also used in other hospital settings where level of consciousness might be altered.

There are three basic elements to the GCS, which are separately assessed and scored into what total score the patient gets. These include eye opening, verbal reaction, and motor function. The scoring is done as is seen in figure 1:

Points	Eye Opening	Verbal Response	Motor Response
1	Doesn't open eyes	Makes no response	No movement
2	Opens to pain stimulus	Is incomprehensible	Decerebrate response
3	Opens to voice command	Speak incoherently	Decorticate response
4	Opens spontaneously	Is confused or disoriented	Broad withdrawal to pain
5		Is fully oriented	Local withdrawal to pain
6			Voluntary movements

In assessing the eye-opening response, a painful stimulus should be given peripherally, such as squeezing the lunula of the fingernail. The patient, in order to score a 4 for eye opening must have both the ability to open their eyes to speech AND spontaneously. The patient does not score a 4 if they have their eyes open but do not have the ability to open and close them with volition.

In assessing the verbal response, there is a gray area between speaking incomprehensibly, speaking incoherently, and being confused or disoriented. Incomprehensive speaking would basically be moaning only, while incoherent speaking involves speaking words that are recognizable but not a pattern of sentence or phrase-utterance. Confused speech involves the ability to answer questions that do not make sense. The person only receives the full five points if they answer questions coherently.

In assessing the motor response, decerebrate posturing involves an extensor response that is exacerbated by pain, while a decorticate response is an exaggerated flexor response to the application of pain. A decorticate response is considered a worse prognostic indicator than a decerebrate response. These are classical responses in patients with severe head injuries. The patient will receive extra points when they are able to indicate where the painful stimulus was given (such as making the appropriate withdrawal response).

The patient is likely to be dead or nearly dead if they receive a score of 3, which is the lowest possible score. Severe impairment is a GCS of less than eight; moderate impairment is a GCS of eight to twelve; mild impairment is a GCS of thirteen or more. Things that impact the scoring without being from a CNS source is the presence of a facial injury that prohibits speech or the presence of an intubated patient that, by definition, cannot speak.

The GCS is a good scale for adults but is not a good scale for semi-conscious children under the age of thirty-six months. Using the adult GCS would yield abnormal test results in even healthy children because they have limited speech. In such cases, there is a pediatric GCS scale used instead for children under the age of three years.

Diagnostics in the Unconscious Patient

The ultimate goal in dealing with the unconscious patient is to identify the underlying cause and treat it. There is no true diagnostic help in stating that the patient is "unconscious" because a wide variety of things could be causing what looks like roughly the same illness. This is where the diagnostic skills of the practitioner are important.

There are three major diagnostic categories that could result in a rapid decline into death in a comatose patient. These include cardiac arrest, airway obstruction, and apnea. These can easily be assessed by checking for a pulse, assessing the degree of spontaneous respirations, and checking to make sure air is moving (which doesn't require a stethoscope necessarily). These are quick and easy evaluations that can be done in a few seconds. It is important to open the airway manually with a head-tilt maneuver or a jaw-thrust maneuver (or an oral or nasal airway). The unconscious patient may not be able to maintain an open airway but this is easily remedied.

There are three things that could result in death within a few minutes to a half an hour. These are not as serious as those listed previous to this but still can result in an early death. These include the patient with an overdose, one with hypoglycemia, and one with increased intracranial pressure and imminent herniation. For this reason, getting a blood sugar is crucial in any unconscious patient as is a quick and focused initial survey.

What should be included in a quick primary survey? These things include the following:

- Pupillary reflex—assesses intracranial pressure
- Corneal reflex
- Extremity movement
- Muscle tone and posturing
- Vital signs
- Capillary refill
- Abdominal palpation
- Overall trauma assessment—looking for obviously traumatized body parts

This type of evaluation takes only about a minute and can lead to the first treatment decision to be made in the care of the unconscious patient. This means that, within a minute, about three things could be diagnosed and treated:

1. **Hypoglycemic coma:** Give one to two amps of intravenous D50W. This will not hurt the patient who is not hypoglycemic but will save the life of a patient severely affected by low blood sugar.
2. **Opioid syndrome:** Give the patient a dose of intravenous naloxone. This will not hurt the patient who does not have opioid syndrome but will save the life of a person with an opioid overdose.
3. **Herniation syndrome:** Elevate the head of the bed, intubate the patient, hyperventilate, and give IV mannitol. This will quickly save the life of a head injury patient if done before the herniation actually happens.

If these things are not a part of the differential diagnosis, there is still a list of things that could kill the patient within the first ten to fifteen minutes of their evaluation. These things can usually be looked out for in the primary survey and include the following:

- Aortic dissection or rupture
- Myocardial infarction
- Hyperkalemia
- Anaphylaxis
- Hypotension
- Arterial blood gas abnormalities

As these things sometimes need more advanced testing than a simple survey, it is a good idea to go beyond the simple survey and do an arterial blood gas measurement and a basic metabolic panel, which will usually involve repeating the blood sugar level, which should be done by means of a glucometer as soon as possible after encountering an unconscious person.

Airway should continually be assessed and, unless the patient awakens quickly, decisions around making a more stable airway should be undertaken—even before an IV is established.

Diagnostically, an EKG and an ultrasound device should be the first tests undertaken. The EKG can rule out an MI or arrhythmia, while an ultrasound can evaluate the abdomen and the aorta.

As the above things are placed into or out of the differential, treatments can be started. Besides oxygen, D50W, and naloxone, which are routine things to start ASAP, the primary survey can lead to several different treatments. Evidence of hypotension can lead to an urgent fluid bolus, followed by blood products. Anaphylaxis symptoms suggest the idea of giving epinephrine. The EKG can suggest an arrhythmia or electrolyte disturbance, which might prompt the giving of calcium gluconate boluses empirically.

The next several things in the differential diagnosis of the unconscious patient involve a group of things that may still kill the patient but won't generally kill the patient for a few hours. These include the following:

- Disorders of metabolism, such as diabetic hyperglycemic disorders, hyponatremia, adrenal insufficiency, and thyroid storm
- Severe abdominal injuries or a ruptured viscus with septicemia
- Necrotizing fasciitis, which can be on any part of the skin
- Status epilepticus
- Alcohol withdrawal syndrome
- Intracranial bleed
- Sepsis/septicemia

Most patients need a CT scan of the head, abdomen, or chest as part of the entire workup. For this reason, they should be completely resuscitated with a definitive airway and relatively stable vital signs. This should be done and blood work should be drawn and may be pending at the time of the CT scan. Antibiotics should be started empirically on everyone with acyclovir started only if viral encephalitis is felt to be the cause. Care should be made to recognize non-convulsive status epilepticus as this requires the same treatment as the actively convulsing patient.

The first few things listed above include those things that can quickly kill the unconscious patient and need urgent ruling in or ruling out. After this is done, a complete differential diagnosis can be made of the various causes of unconsciousness. This involves a much longer list and includes things that will shortly kill the patient and things that may take hours to days to be deadly if not treated. The full differential includes the following:

- Alcohol poisoning/overdose
- Metabolic acidosis
- Hepatic encephalopathy with hyperammonemia
- Arrhythmia
- Endocrine disorder like myxedema or adrenal crisis
- Electrolyte abnormality
- Anoxic encephalopathy
- Septicemia/severe infection
- Hypoxia

- Drug overdose
- Uremic encephalopathy
- Traumatic brain injury

You should have this checklist handy in the emergency department or on your smart phone in order to make sure all the possibilities for a comatose state that can quickly kill the patient are consciously looked at and ruled in or out. This will make for a rapid diagnosis and definitely treatment (if there is one).

The empiric treatments that should be given upon encountering any unconscious patient before all tests are back include a fluid bolus, glucose as D50W, naloxone, antibiotic, thyroxine, benzodiazepines (for non-convulsive status epilepticus), and dexamethasone for adrenal insufficiency.

Key Takeaways

- An unconscious patient has a complete or nearly complete lack of awareness of their surroundings.
- There is a gradient from full consciousness, through confusion and stupor, to eventual full unconsciousness.
- The Glasgow Coma Scale is a reliable and objective measurement of levels of consciousness in patients with altered mental states.
- There are things in the differential diagnosis of unconsciousness that need to be urgently addressed and things that can wait until a full assessment is done.

Quiz

1. What term best describes a state of altered mental status?
   a. Disorientation
   b. Confusion
   c. Stupor
   d. All of the above

Answer: d. All of the above represent terms that can be used to describe an altered mental status. They can be used interchangeably.

2. Which of the following causes of unconsciousness isn't related to hypoperfusion of the brain?
   a. Hypoglycemia
   b. Dehydration
   c. Arrhythmia
   d. Acute blood loss

Answer: a. Of the above choices, only hypoglycemia results in unconsciousness that is not directly related to hypoperfusion of the brain, while the other causes of unconsciousness are directly related to decreased brain perfusion.

3. Which sensory dysfunction is not a criterion for being unconscious?
   a. Lack of ability to respond to visual stimuli
   b. Lack of ability to respond to pain stimuli
   c. Lack of ability to respond to auditory stimuli
   d. Lack of ability to respond to light touch

Answer: b. Lack of ability to respond to pain stimuli is not a necessary criterion for being unconscious as unconscious patients may still reflexively respond to a painful stimulus.

4. For what reason might you place an unconscious patient on their left side?
   a. To maximize blood flow to the heart.
   b. To encourage spontaneous breathing.
   c. To protect the cervical and lumbar spine.
   d. To protect their airway from possible aspiration.

Answer: d. The main reason why an unconscious person should be kept on their side is to protect their airway from aspiration, should they vomit or bring up secretions.

5. A special situation exists when a known diabetic has an altered mental status. What is the correct approach?
   a. Give them oral glucose solution or an oral sugar tablet to restore consciousness.
   b. Give oral glucose supplement or something sweet only if they are conscious.
   c. Give oral glucose supplement or something sweet only if they are oriented.
   d. Obtain a stat blood sugar level with a glucometer before proceeding with hypoglycemia treatment.

Answer: b. The patient with diabetes should receive oral glucose or something sweet but only if they are conscious. They do not have to be oriented and a blood sugar does not have to be obtained before doing this.

6. You have witnessed a middle-aged man become unconscious after choking on a piece of meat. What is the first step?
   a. Look for a loose foreign body in the oropharynx.
   b. Sit the patient up and do the Heimlich maneuver.
   c. Perform chest compressions.
   d. Start artificial respirations.

Answer: c. The goal of doing chest compressions in this type of situation is to attempt to dislodge the foreign object. Doing chest compressions will increase the intrathoracic pressure and may dislodge the item without having to do anything else.

7. The patient with a head injury does not open his eyes to painful stimuli. What GCS score for eye opening do you give him?
   a. One
   b. Two
   c. Three
   d. Four

Answer: a. The person who does not open his eyes to painful stimuli should receive a GCS score for eye opening of one.

8. The patient you are evaluating has a GCS score of 13. What level of CNS impairment do they have?
   a. Severe
   b. Moderate
   c. Minor
   d. No impairment

Answer: c. The patient with a GCS score of thirteen is said to have a minor GCS impairment.

9. Which is not considered something that could result in death in a couple of minutes in an unconscious patient?
   a. Apnea
   b. Cardiac arrest
   c. Airway obstruction
   d. Increased intracranial pressure

Answer: d. The three main things that could result in death immediately in an unconscious patient include apnea, cardiac arrest, and airway obstruction. Increased intracranial pressure is not likely to result in sudden death.

10. Which of the following should not be given empirically to an unconscious patient until a complete diagnosis is established?
    a. Tissue plasminogen activator
    b. Glucose
    c. Antibiotics
    d. Naloxone

Answer: Glucose, antibiotics, and naloxone (among others) should be given empirically; however, there should be evidence for a need to give tissue plasminogen activator as this can cause more harm than good if the diagnosis of a clot hasn't been made first.

Chapter 2: CPR Basics for Adults

The care of the critically-ill patient begins with a thorough knowledge of adult cardiorespiratory resuscitation or CPR. The exact way this procedure is carried out has changed over the years as new research becomes available. A basic and indelible knowledge of CPR should be the cornerstone of your education in basic and advanced life support because you will not always be in a well-staffed medical facility when you encounter the patient needing cardiorespiratory resuscitation.

Preparation for CPR

It is difficult to think about preparedness for CPR because it usually represents an acute medical situation that needs urgent action. Still, there are things the provider needs to think about in advance of actually performing CPR.

The patient needing CPR is generally completely unconscious, so you don't need to worry about anesthesia or about hurting them as they will not be responsive to pain. CPR carries the risk of pain secondary to rib or sternal fractures but these tend not to become symptomatic until the patient wakes up and is resuscitated. There are few complications of these types of fractures, except for the occasional pneumothorax or cardiac contusion from excessive application of chest compressions.

You may not have any access to equipment when you do CPR in the field; however, there are inflatable facial masks that can be carried in a packet on one's key chain to prevent disease secondary to mouth-to-mouth resuscitation. If possible, gloves should be worn as you may come in contact with the patient's blood in a trauma situation.

Up until now, no reported cases of disease transmission have become public knowledge so that even without protective mask or gloves, CPR should be able to be safely done in just about any setting, particularly if the patient is not a trauma patient who is actively bleeding.

Some EMS teams and hospitals use a mechanical chest compression device, which should be tested and calibrated before being used on the patient because the device delivers different levels of thrust depending on the setting. It should be noted that there is no mechanical advantage to using this type of compressor over delivering high-quality manual compressions. Some studies have shown an advantage but this has not been a universal finding in all studies.

If you happen to be an ACLS provider (Advanced Cardiac Life Support provider), you may opt to put in an endotracheal tube in order to provide better ventilation for the patient. The main advantage of doing this over a bag-mask valve device or mouth-to-mouth resuscitation is that it protects the airway from both secretions and any vomiting that might happen. It should be performed only by a trained ACLS provider as putting an ET tube in incorrectly can have disastrous complications.

The final device that you might want to have ready for use is the external cardiac defibrillator. These are available for use in many public places and should be strongly considered to be used anytime there is an out-of-hospital cardiac arrest. These devices are on standby for anybody to use but they must be retrieved by a bystander and used as soon as it is able to read a shockable rhythm as rapid defibrillation probably has the greatest impact over survival when compared to all other parameters in basic CPR with the best neurological and overall outcome.

CPR Basics

The first step in actually doing CPR is positioning. Make sure that the patient you are about to do CPR on is supine and on a relatively hard surface. It may mean moving the patient away from a couch or mattress and onto a hard surface, such as the floor. Compressions are ineffective when performed on a soft surface. The floor is also an advantage because it affords the provider a chance to be a great deal above the victim when performing chest compressions. A patient on a table or other high surface may be too high for effective compressions.

Figure 2 shows the different steps in CPR:

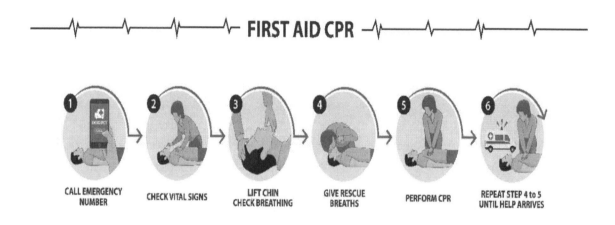

Figure 2

The goal of CPR is to maintain oxygenation through chest compressions and ventilations until a rhythm that is survivable can be restored. Chest compressions and ventilations are done along with an automatic external defibrillator (If available) until EMS arrives, the patient awakens or resumes spontaneous cardiac and respiratory activity, or until the provide becomes exhausted.

The fact of the matter is that CPR alone on a patient who has sustained an out-of-hospital cardiac arrest does not have a good survival rate. The average survival rate of such an arrest is about ten percent, with survival that includes good neurological function being about eight percent. About a third of all victims who have a witnessed arrest will survive their event. Patients need to ultimately receive some sort of advanced live support to survive, which will be topics of another chapter.

Chest Compressions in CPR

Chest compressions in adults should be done at a rate comparable to a normal person's heart rate under stressful conditions, which is about a hundred compressions per minute. The provision of CPR involves three parts, with compressions being the first thing that is done on the patient who has arrested. Bystander CPR (in an untrained individual) should involve chest compressions only as the other components have not been found to add to the survival rate.

Figure 3 indicates what chest compressions look like:

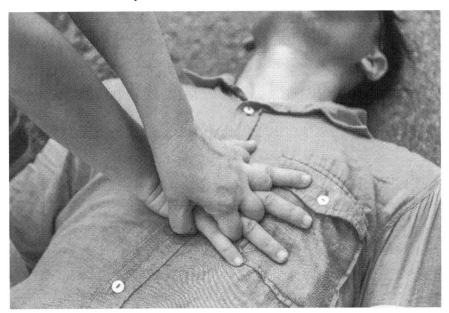

Figure 3

Thirty chest compressions should be done upon determining the pulseless status of the patient. After this, the head-tilt, chin-lift maneuver should be done to open the airway. This can only be done on a patient not suspected of having a cervical spine injury and involves slightly tilting back the head and opening the airway by lifting the chin. An obstruction should be ruled out by looking in the airway before doing ventilations.

When doing chest compressions, the provider should place the heel of the hand on the lower third of the sternum with the opposite hand placed on top so that the fingers interlace. Elbows are kept straight and the provider should lean so that he or she is directly above the patient's heart. The compression should result in a displacement of the sternum by at least two inches before releasing and allowing for chest recoil.

Each set of compressions proceeds for thirty compressions total or for about twenty-three seconds. This is a rate of about a hundred compressions per second. The key is to push hard and fast without leaning on the patient so that full recoil can be accomplished between compressions. After the thirty compressions, two breaths should be given. This provides about six to eight breaths per minute. If two providers are available, the ventilator should do about eight to ten breaths a minute.

If there are multiple resuscitators, good quality CPR is best maintained when the providers switch places or swap out every two to three minutes because giving chest compressions Is very tiring and cannot be sustained for much longer than three minutes before the compressions are less effective.

Ventilations in CPR

Ventilations are only done with providers trained in the full CPR technique. This usually means that only a healthcare provider should do ventilations; however, a certified layperson may be able to accomplish this without difficulty. A bag-valve-mask device (BVM) is preferred over mouth-to-mouth resuscitation provided the person giving the respirations is trained in using this device.

In giving mouth-to-mouth resuscitation, the nostrils should be pinched off with the head slightly tilted back. The provider makes a seal with his or her mouth completely over the victim's mouth. The provider delivers a breath that both lasts for about a second and causes a visible rise in the victim's chest wall.

If a bag-valve-mask is available and the provider is trained in its use, the mask should be placed over the victim's mouth and nose, with the cushioned part of the mask forming a tight seal around the individual's oral and nasal area. The bag should be squeezed firmly for one second, delivering a minimum of five hundred milliliters of air into the patient's lungs.

Indications for CPR

CPR should be done without delay in any person who is found to be both pulseless and unconscious for any reason. The loss of an effective pulse can happen for a variety of reasons, the vast majority of which are cardiac in origin and related to a nonperfusing rhythm. Those arrhythmias that do not generally profuse the body well include these:

- Pulseless bradycardia—there may be a beat on the rhythm strip but the cardiac output is ineffective and unable to cause a pulse.
- Asystole—the rhythm strip would show the absence of a pulse or any cardiac impulse.
- Pulseless electrical activity (PEA)—the rhythm strip may show just about anything but there is no effective cardiac output so the patient is pulseless.
- Pulseless ventricular tachycardia (VT)—this can be a rhythm with a pulse but often, the rate is so fast, the heart cannot fill and the cardiac output is inefficient.
- Ventricular fibrillation (VF)—the patient's heart is fibrillating and there is no clear QRS complex on the rhythm strip.

CPR needs to start even before a rhythm strip is obtained as the absence of a pulse should be identification enough that the patient has one of the above rhythms happening. If there is an automatic external defibrillator available, it should be applied and charges while CPR is ongoing. The defibrillator will determine if the rhythm is shockable and will tell everyone to "clear" the patient while the shock is being delivered. CPR should begin as soon as the shock is given unless a pulsatile state is achieved by the shock.

According to experts in the field of CPR and resuscitation, there are some guidelines that should be followed in giving CPR in the field:

- It may be appropriate to withhold the process of CPR in cases where there is a victim who has sustained penetrating or blunt trauma and who is obviously dead or will not survive.
- All non-traumatized individuals should have CPR unless there is a clear DNR order or living will stating that no resuscitative efforts should be made.
- If a trauma patient is treated with CPR who had an unwitnessed event and who sustained severe trauma may be limited to thirty minutes of CPR before stopping.
- Anyone who had a drowning event with hypothermia or who had a lightning strike injury should have CPR performed.
- When the circumstances of the unconsciousness are in doubt, CPR should be started until the patient arrives and is evaluated at the emergency department.

The only reason not to perform CPR on a patient is if they have an advanced directive or DNR order that is clearly established and that indicates the victim's desire not to be resuscitated after a cardiac arrest. The only, far secondary, reason not to do CPR is if a licensed healthcare provider determines that intervening with CPR would not help save the patient's life. This can be done prior to starting CPR or after CPR has already begun. It is rare that an advanced directive or DNR order is clearly established before starting CPR.

Complications of CPR

There are two main complications of CPR. The first is fractures of either the sternum or ribcage because of aggressive chest compressions. This is relatively uncommon unless the cardiac arrest happens in an elderly person with osteoporosis or who is extremely frail.

The second complication is called "gastric insufflation" and happens when the ventilations are given without an endotracheal tube, which effectively seals off the airway from the gastrointestinal tract. If a person has had a prolonged period of CPR without an endotracheal tube, they may need a post-arrest nasogastric (NG) tube to relieve the pressure that could cause post-arrest vomiting once the patient awakens.

ACLS versus BLS

In most cases, an out-of-hospital cardiac arrest means there is no equipment and CPR plus or minus the automatic external defibrillator (AED) are the only options. When an advanced provider is there, such as an EMS team with an ambulance, the focus shifts from BLS (Basic Life Support) to ACLS (Advanced Cardiac Life Support). In a trauma patient with EMS services activated, protocols for ATLS (Advanced Trauma Life Support) are activated.

Both ACLS and ATLS differ from BLS in that there is continual ECG monitoring, defibrillation (which can be in BLS as well if an AED is present, drug interventions, and invasive airway techniques. In ACLS, there are protocols available for all rhythms and situations. No longer is atropine recommended for PEA or asystole and no longer is cricoid pressure recommended with CPR.

Key Takeaways

- BLS in adults may involve chest compressions only (in laypeople CPR) or a combination of chest compressions and ventilations (in provider-associated BLS).
- Chest compressions go at a rate of 100 beats per minute for thirty compressions before two rescue breaths are given.
- CPR should only be held in a trauma patient who is not expected to survive or who appears dead, or in a patient who has a known DNR declaration documented.

Quiz

1. What is the main advantage to using a mechanical compressor in CPR?
    a. It delivers faster compressions than manual CPR.
    b. It can give deeper compressions than manual CPR.
    c. There is better neurological outcome when using a mechanical compressor.
    d. There has been no proof that mechanical compressors are superior to good manual CPR.

Answer: d. There have been a few studies showing mechanical compression to be better than manual CPR but this hasn't been borne out in all studies so it is not considered superior to good manual CPR technique.

2. What is considered the main advantage of using an endotracheal tube to deliver respirations in CPR over any other method?
    a. It can be done with facial trauma when mouth-to-mouth can't be done.
    b. It protects the airway from vomiting and secretions being aspirated.
    c. It offers no advantage over doing mouth-to-mouth resuscitation.
    d. There is less provider fatigue with this method.

Answer: b. The main advantage of using an endotracheal tube to deliver respirations in CPR is that it protects the airway from vomiting and aspiration of secretions, which is something that cannot be done with mouth-to-mouth resuscitation or other ways of delivering respirations.

3. What aspect of basic CPR is important to incorporate for the best possible neurological outcome and survival?
    a. Automatic external defibrillation as soon as possible
    b. Endotracheal intubation to be performed as soon as possible

c. Using a mechanical compressor for chest compressions

d. Having IV access as soon as possible

Answer: a. The automatic external defibrillator has offered patients the best chance for an acceptable neurological outcome and enhanced overall survival when compared to other aspects of CPR.

4. Which is not a part of the standard part of a provider-based CPR protocol?
   a. Chest compressions
   b. Airway opening
   c. Ventilations
   d. Intravenous access

Answer: d. Chest compressions, airway opening/management, and ventilations are all a part of provider-based CPR in its fullest form. Intravenous access is not a part of this process as the equipment to do this would not be available in an out-of-hospital setting.

5. You are advising a middle-aged woman who has just witnessed her husband have an episode of unconsciousness. She says he is not breathing and has no pulse. You have access to 911 services already. What should you tell her to do first?
   a. Deliver thirty seconds of chest compressions at a hundred compressions per minute.
   b. Clean out the mouth and clear out any foreign body that might be there.
   c. Deliver two quick breaths, followed by chest compressions at a hundred beats per minute.
   d. Start artificial respirations at twenty breaths a minute for thirty seconds.

Answer: a. A non-healthcare provider should do compressions only, starting with thirty seconds of compressions to see what happens. Ventilations are not recommended for bystander CPR in the untrained individual.

6. How many compressions are done before opening the airway in a provider-based CPR routine?
   a. Thirty seconds' worth
   b. A minutes' worth
   c. Thirty total compressions
   d. One hundred total compressions

Answer: c. Thirty total compressions should be done before performing the head tilt-chin lift maneuver.

7. How long should one breath take in giving mouth-to-mouth ventilations?
   a. One second
   b. Two seconds
   c. Three seconds
   d. Four seconds

Answer: a. A good ventilation should take only about a second to perform and should involve a visible rise in the patient's chest wall.

8. What is not considered a common pulseless rhythm requiring urgent CPR?
   a. Ventricular fibrillation
   b. Asystole
   c. Supraventricular tachycardia
   d. Pulseless electrical activity (PEA)

Answer: c. All of the above are considered common pulseless rhythms with the exception of supraventricular tachycardia, which is usually symptomatic but not always pulseless unless it is very fast.

9. About how many milliliters of air are delivered per breath with a bag-valve-mask?
   a. 250 milliliters
   b. 500 milliliters
   c. 750 milliliters
   d. 1000 milliliters

Answer: b. On average, about 500 milliliters of air at a minimum should be delivered to the chest per ventilation with a BVM.

10. What feature of resuscitation can be found in both BLS protocol and ACLS protocol?
    a. Drug interventions
    b. Endotracheal tube resuscitation
    c. Defibrillation
    d. ECG monitoring

Answer: c. Defibrillation can be an aspect of either BLS or ACLS, while the other choices are necessarily only seen in ACLS protocols.

Chapter 3: CPR Basics for Children and Infants

This chapter involves the special circumstances that exist when giving CPR to children and infants. Rather than a cardiac cause, most cardiac arrests in children are not due to primary heart disease but to other problems. This will be covered as part of the chapter. The basics of how to do quality CPR will be discussed as well as how an AED should be used in pediatric CPR.

Pediatric Cardiac Arrests

At least five thousand children in the US have an atraumatic cardiac arrest in an out-of-hospital setting. Factors that play into survival from this serious medical problem include the physical environment, any preexisting health conditions the child has, the initial rhythm strip discovered, the quality of CPR and ACLS services, and the duration of lack of blood flow before resuscitation begins.

Most out-of-hospital cardiac arrests in children are not actually related to a cardiac event. In fact, these types of arrests are twice as likely to be secondary to something that is noncardiac in origin when compared to pediatric heart disease. Fortunately, this means that the outcomes are much better after an out-of-hospital event than people older than 18 years of age.

Causes of pediatric out-of-hospital cardiac arrests include the following:

- Asphyxia—Sudden infant death syndrome, drowning, hanging, foreign body inhalation, smoke inhalations, central apnea, or acute respiratory disease.
- Circulatory shock—Sepsis, trauma, congenital heart disease, arrhythmia, dehydration, or myocarditis.
- Neurological dysfunction—seizures or increased intracranial pressure
- Toxic ingestion—which can be a medication or household toxic ingestion

The way to survival for a child who has suffered a cardiorespiratory arrest includes five major elements. These include the following:

- Prevention of a cardiac arrest
- Effective and early CPR
- Early call for help
- Implementation of advanced life support for children
- Aggressive post-resuscitation care

Surprisingly, effective bystander CPR is one of the most crucial factors for increasing the survival of the child who has sustained a cardiac arrest outside of a medical facility. Unfortunately, only one third of children actually receive the necessary CPR after an arrest, giving precious minutes away in which the child hypoxic while waiting for EMS services.

Figure 4 shows CPR on an infant:

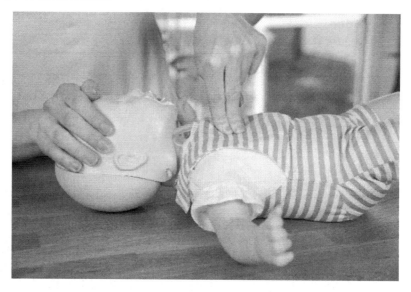

Figure 4

The recommendation for laypeople is to do chest compressions only as this has been found to be just as effective as chest compressions plus ventilation support. Why is this the case? There are three major reasons why this works:

- There is enough oxygen in the lungs to exchange with carbon dioxide in the lungs for up to fifteen minutes after the arrest.
- Gasping happens with CPR, which facilitates gas exchange.
- Chest recoil allows for air to enter the lungs, adding to oxygenation.

On the other hand, most cardiac arrests in children come from an asphyxic event, meaning that the child is already hypoxic and oxygen-depleted at the time they have their arrest. Add to this the fact that gasping tends not to occur in children who are already oxygen deprived and you find that it is actually more effective and improves survival if both chest compressions and ventilations are given rather than chest compressions alone.

Even with this knowledge, it is still recommended that CPR for bystanders involves only chest compressions because it is too complex for the bystander to determine the cause of an arrest in a child and doing compressions and ventilations together is too complex when compared to doing chest compressions alone. In fact, the mnemonic CAB is recommended, which stands for compressions-airway-breathing. This is the order that CPR should ideally happen in children. This is because flow is necessary to get the partially oxygenated blood to the tissues and must be initiated first.

It is crucial to have high quality CPR, which is identified as compressing the chest about a third of the chest diameter, fast and uninterrupted compressions, and minimal ventilation. This maximizes the survival rate. Compression depth, unfortunately, is often inadequate, even by trained health professionals. The goal should be more than a hundred compressions per minute as this restores spontaneous circulation with better chances of recovery. Leaning on the chest during the relaxation phase will decrease the chest recoil and is not recommended. Unfortunately, it often happens; however, too low a depth of compressions is the biggest mistake people make in doing CPR in children.

No one knows the optimal dose of energy to be delivered per defibrillation in children. Ideally, about two to four Joules per kilogram should be given as a first dose. Because automated external defibrillators are highly sensitive in picking up a shockable rhythm, they are recommended for the pediatric population as well as the adult population. Even though the dose given is higher than desirable for this age group, giving a shock that is too strong is better than giving no shock at all.

This is not the case, however, in children under the age of one year of age. The automated external defibrillator will send too much energy to the child receiving bystander CPR, so manual and controllable defibrillation is recommended in children under this age.

Pediatric BLS Guidelines

Recent guidelines have pointed toward the mnemonic "CAB" rather than the historical pattern of "ABC" because this has been found to be a better approach than previous approaches to pediatric CPR. Upon finding a child who is unresponsive and pulseless, the first thing that should be done is to shout for help. A second person should ideally activate the EMS system and gets any available automated external defibrillator (AED), while the first person stays with the victim. A mobile phone should be used to activate the EMS system if the individual is alone with the child.

The major difference between the initiation of CPR with a healthcare provider versus a layperson is the finding of a pulse. A pulse should be assessed over a ten second period of time in an apneic child if the person is a healthcare provider, while a layperson should simply observe that the child is not breathing before starting compressions.

The recommended compression rate for children is about a hundred to a hundred twenty compressions per minute at a depth of one third of the AP diameter of the chest. If the provider determines that the child has a pulse, respirations are initiated at a rate of about twelve to twenty breaths per minute, which is about one every three to five seconds. Chest compressions should be started if the pulse is ever found to dip below sixty beats per minute. If the pulse is less than sixty and the child appears well-perfused, compressions do not have to be done. A pulse should be rechecked every two minutes while CPR is ongoing.

If there is only one rescuer trained in child CPR, there should be thirty chest compressions and then two breaths per CPR cycle. If there are two rescuers trained in CPR, the cycle should consist of fifteen compressions and then two breaths. If there is one rescuer and no cell phone, CPR should happen for two minutes before quickly leaving to get an AED and activating the EMS system. The AED should be attached to the patient as soon as it arrives so it can begin detecting a rhythm.

If a shockable rhythm is detected, the rescuers need to stay clear of the patient and should wait for the shock to be delivered. The pulse should not be checked right after the shock but should be assessed after doing another two minutes of CPR and allowing the AED to detect the rhythm. CPR should be continued until EMS arrives or until the patient shows some motor movement. Of course, if the provider becomes exhausted and cannot continue, CPR can be stopped.

When doing compressions in children, the depth of the compressions is about a third that of the AP diameter of the child's chest. This is about four centimeters in infants, five centimeters in children, and five centimeters in adolescents. At no time should it exceed about six centimeters. There should be complete recoil after each compression and the provider shouldn't lean on the patient, which will adversely affect recoil.

Some key things to remember about doing CPR on children between the ages of one and eighteen include the following:

- The pulse needs to be checked at the carotid artery.
- The compressions should be done over the lower half of the sternum
- About five centimeters is the recommended depth of compressions.
- There should be adequate recoil after each compression.
- The compression rate should be a hundred to one hundred twenty beats per minute.
- The person doing the compression needs to be rotated out every two minutes in order to avoid fatigue.
- Interruptions in compressions should last no longer than ten seconds (which is the time it takes to assess the pulse.
- Excessive ventilation should be avoided with respirations to go on at a rate of twelve to twenty breaths per minute.

With infants, the biggest difference in doing CPR is that the pulse is assessed at the brachial artery rather than the carotid artery (as is done in children and adults). The rest of the protocol is the same as is found in children. Another difference is in the use of the AED, which is not recommended for infants as they should have a manually-driven automated external defibrillator with infant-appropriate pads.

The airway should be opened in all cases of childhood CPR. In children over the age of one, the head should be tilted and the chin lifted forward. In infants, their head should be placed in a "sniffing position" to maximize airflow. If a cervical spine injury is suspected, just the jaw thrust maneuver should be done with the head kept in a neutral position.

Key Takeaways

- Child CPR progresses with the CAB protocol versus the ABC protocol that was once used.
- The major causes of cardiac arrest in children is secondary to non-cardiac reasons.
- CPR should go on with a single rescuer at thirty compressions for every two breaths.
- If two providers are present, the cycle should be fifteen compressions for every two breaths.
- The AED cannot be used in infants but can be used in children over the age of one year.

Quiz

1. What is not considered a major factor in the outcome of a pediatric cardiac arrest?
   a. The physical environment the arrest occurs in
   b. The preexisting condition of the child
   c. The age of the child
   d. The quality of the CPR

Answer: c. The above choices represent major factors in the outcome of a pediatric cardiac arrest, except for the age of the child, which isn't a major factor.

2. What cause of pediatric cardiac arrest is not secondary to circulatory collapse?
   a. Upper respiratory infection
   b. Sepsis
   c. Arrhythmia
   d. Trauma

Answer: a. An upper respiratory infection is a cause of a pediatric cardiac arrest but does not cause circulatory collapse.

3. What would the least likely cause of an out-of-hospital cardiac arrest in a child?
   a. Drowning
   b. SIDS
   c. Trauma
   d. Coronary artery disease

Answer: d. Coronary artery disease is not considered a major cause of an out-of-hospital cardiac arrest, while the others are common causes of an out of hospital cardiac arrest in a child.

4. What is the biggest mistake made in doing child CPR?
   a. Doing chest compressions too quickly.
   b. Doing chest compressions too slowly.
   c. Compressing the chest too little.
   d. Doing too many ventilations.

Answer: c. All of the above mistakes can be made by persons doing CPR in children; however, applying too little force during compressions is considered the most common mistake that people make during CPR efforts.

5. What is the recommended initial shock dose in defibrillating a child with an AED?
   a. Two to four Joules per kilogram
   b. The AED shocks at a set energy level, even in children.
   c. Two hundred Joules
   d. One hundred Joules

Answer: b. The AED shocks at a set energy level that cannot be controlled, even in children.

6. What should the initial step be in doing CPR in a child who has been found to be unconscious in the field by a layperson?
   a. Check the pulse
   b. Begin cardiac compressions at 100 beats per minute
   c. Begin artificial respiration for five breaths
   d. Assess that the child is not breathing

Answer: d. Before starting CPR, the layperson should assess that the child is not breathing. They do not need to check the pulse as this has been deemed too complex for the layperson to perform. Chest compressions should start after it has been determined that the patient is not breathing.

7. How long should a single rescuer do CPR on a child before activating the EMS system (even if it means briefly leaving the child)?
   a. One minute
   b. Two minutes
   c. Five minutes
   d. Ten minutes

Answer: b. CPR should go on for two minutes without activating the EMS system before the single rescuer leaves the child to activate the system.

8. What should happen next after the AED performs a shock in a child undergoing two-person CPR?
   a. Recheck the pulse as soon as the shock is over.
   b. Give two rescue breaths and then check the pulse.
   c. Do chest compressions only for thirty seconds and then recheck the pulse.
   d. Do chest compressions and ventilations per recommendations for two minutes before checking the pulse.

Answer: d. After the AED has shocked the patient, the two-person team needs to restart CPR per protocol for two minutes before checking the pulse and allowing the AED to detect the rhythm.

9. What is not considered a proper end-point for bystander CPR in children?
   a. The EMS system arrives to take over.

b. The patient is visibly moving.

c. The CPR has continued for thirty minutes without restoration of the pulse.

d. The provider is exhausted and cannot continue.

Answer: c. There is no time limit as to when to stop CPR on a child except if EMS arrives, the patient moves, or the provider fatigues to the point of exhaustion.

10. What is the main difference in using the AED in infants versus using the AED in adults?

a. There is no difference as shocking too much is better than not shocking at all.

b. The AED should be set to deliver half the dose that is given to adults.

c. The AED should be used at full strength but with smaller AED pads.

d. The AED should not be used and manually-driven defibrillation should take place instead.

Answer: d. In infants, the AED should not be used and a manually-driven defibrillator should take place instead as the Joules give would be too high for an infant.

Chapter 4: Automated External Defibrillator Use

So far, we have covered the topics of basic CPR for both adults and children who have sustained a cardiac arrest. As part of this process, an automated external defibrillator was discussed as it has been shown to improve survival rate of the patient suffering from an out-of-hospital cardiac arrest. In this chapter, we will focus more on the automated external defibrillator or AED and will attempt to explain how it is used best in the field setting.

AED Basics

The first studies on giving electrical shocks to correct ventricular fibrillation was done on dogs. Researchers discovered that, if dogs were defibrillated within thirty seconds of inducing ventricular fibrillation, the success rate was 98 percent. If the researches waited two minutes to give the electrical shock, however, the success rate dropped to 27 percent. This research eventually gave rise to the idea that, if defibrillation can be done rapidly enough, people could actually survive an out-of-hospital cardiac arrest. The idea was conceived of having automatic external defibrillators or AEDs on the scene to shock patients with a shockable rhythm as soon as possible.

Figure 5 shows an AED on a CPR dummy:

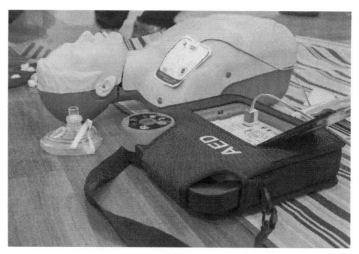

Figure 5

The survival rate for ventricular fibrillation after having an AED placed and utilized is about 30 percent (however, the actual rate depends on the study used). This compares to a survival rate with CPR alone in patients with ventricular fibrillation of about six percent. In theory, the survival rate could be even higher if the public had close access to an AED and if the AED were to be applied within several seconds of the arrest. Sadly, only about 10-15 percent of out-of-hospital arrests happen in a public place where AEDs are generally placed.

Defibrillators were first put in practice in the 1920s because of a large increase in the number of deaths secondary to electrical shocks. Cardiac paddles were first used with the first successful defibrillation in humans happening in 1947. The first person successfully defibrillated was a fourteen-year-old male who developed a non-perfusing rhythm during open heart surgery. This was not an external defibrillation; however. The first external defibrillation didn't happen until 1956.

Research in the 1960s focused on whether DC (direct current) defibrillation was better than AC (alternating current) defibrillation for defibrillation. It was at this time that it was first determined that DC current was superior to AC current. It was safer than AC current and was more effective in turning a person with ventricular fibrillation to normal sinus rhythm. It was in 1966 that the first ambulance-based defibrillation was found to be successful. The first defibrillation that was performed solely by EMTs was reported to have occurred in 1969.

It was in the 1970s and early 1980s that the first companies came out with usable defibrillators for use in the field. The first device was heavy at twenty-eight pounds and made use of an oral and precordial electrode instead of the precordial pads used today. The ability to use transcutaneous pacing was first developed in the early 1980s as well. Police officers and other first responders were trained to use these devices in the early half of the 1980s; however, the AED wasn't available in public places until later.

In the early 1990s, the use by laypeople of AEDs was approved by the FDA with legislation making it safe to use the device without risk of being sued for liability being put in place at about the same time. AED training was first included in basic CPR courses starting in 1999. By 2004, the first AEDs to be sold for home use were allowed without a doctor's prescription. In 2004, it was mandated that AEDs be on all passenger-carrying airlines in the US. Since that time, AEDs have been successfully used in airports, stadiums, schools, malls, and casinos.

Early models of AEDs necessitated the use of an oral/epigastric electrode along with an external chest electrode. Now, AEDs use a right sternal border and cardiac apex pad that serve to both monitor the arrhythmia, detect a shockable rhythm, and defibrillate. They can tell the user if the contact is poor, when the machine is ready to defibrillate, when the user should check for a pulse, when patient motion is detected, and when a shockable rhythm is present. It can also say when a non-shockable rhythm is present.

The first AEDs would respond to a heart rate greater than 150 beats per minute and a QRS amplitude higher than 0.15 mm. Now, the ECG rhythm is detected by several different methods. Not only is the rate and QRS amplitude measured, but the QRS slope, density, and morphology is assessed. Every 2-4 seconds, the machine assesses the rhythm and if an abnormal rhythm that is shockable is detected over three separate times (in a row), the AED will be ready to deliver a shock. The sensitivity in assessing accurately the presence of ventricular fibrillation is about 76-96 percent with a specificity of about 100 percent.

Monophasic defibrillation will deliver a shock only in one direction. Biphasic defibrillation involves giving a charge in one direction for half the time and in the opposite direction for the other half of the time. Monophasic charges require higher energy levels so, for this reason, most internal defibrillators are biphasic, and more external defibrillators are becoming biphasic because it takes less time to charge and because the battery life is longer.

AEDs were compared to manual defibrillators as to their successfulness. The rates of admission and survival to discharge were equivalent for either type of defibrillation. Another study, in 1988, showed that the use of the AED by non-first-responders was only 3.3 minutes, compared to 8.8 minutes with EMT-mediated defibrillation. There was, in this study, a higher survival to discharge rate in the patients who were resuscitated with AEDs compared to waiting for the EMTs or paramedics (30 percent versus 19 percent).

Results of studies on the success of defibrillation with AEDs has been somewhat inconsistent with some studies showing no advantage of having AEDs available for public use. Some of the reason why AEDs were found to be questionable include the fact that the survival rate for unwitnessed arrests is very small, even with AEDs available. What this means is that, if the arrest is unwitnessed, it doesn't matter if an AED is nearby because the time to shock may, in fact, be much longer than the three-minute response time found in those arrests that are witnessed. The key factor in survival with defibrillation is the time to defibrillation and not the actual device used.

Further research on AED use found that about 17 percent of patients needed another defibrillation after the initial shock. Patients who convert the first time have about the same survival rate as patients who need to be defibrillated a second time. Again, the time to defibrillation is crucial so that fully automated devices that will deliver the shock faster are superior to semi-automated devices that require some input from the provider in order to deliver a shock.

Precautions when using an AED

The AED should only be applied to patients who are pulseless and the assessment by the AED needs to happen only if the patient is pulseless. Using the AED on a patient who already has a pulse could be dangerous and could result in the patient developing a rhythm that is worse than the rhythm they had in the first place.

To prevent being accidentally shocked, the unit shouldn't analyze the rhythm while CPR is being performed. Most AEDs have a CPR detector or "motion detector" so it won't search out the rhythm until the CPR is halted. AEDs shouldn't be used on seizing patients and should be used cautiously in moving vehicles because it will not work when the patient is moving.

The chest does not have to be shaved before placing the electrode but it should be dried off if wet. Minor skin lacerations or wet spots could lead to local skin burns and uneven defibrillation. Nitroglycerin patches must be removed as they might cause an explosion. If the AED says "check electrode" when the electrodes seem properly placed, the electrodes should be replaced as they are probably defective.

AEDs may need to be reprogrammed if they do not have the current American Heart Association Defibrillation Guidelines. If the AED is an older model, it needs to be assessed to see what programming it has and it should be reprogrammed if there are changes in the Guidelines. Always check the FDA recall website and remove the AED from use if it has been recalled for any reason.

AEDs are probably ineffective in highly rural areas where the chance of a witnessed arrest is low. It is probably effective if placed on a plane, in airports, in high traffic areas, and anytime the response rate for a first responder is less than 4-6 minutes. Shocking past 4-6 minutes with an AED is not likely to be helpful to the patient. Wiring for AEDs should be compatible with the wiring used by EMS and paramedic services.

Public Access Defibrillation

This is also referred to as PAD. It has been found to be most effective when placed in senior centers, universities, casinos, health clubs, stadiums airports, and airplanes, where there are high risk patients and where the arrest is likely to be witnessed. It is mandated to be in place in airplanes but not in any of the other areas.

Using the AED

Each AED is slightly different but most are designed to have basically the same rules and instructions so that no one who is trained in AED-assisted CPR needs to read any instruction manual before being able to use the AED. As discussed, the AED is definitely successful when used on a child or adult weighing a minimum of 55 pounds. It can be used on younger children weighing less than this but will deliver an impulse that is higher than is recommended for that size. For anyone older than one year of age, however, a shock that is too high is better than not getting a shock at all. AEDs for adults should not be used in children under the age of one year.

The steps to using an AED include the following:

- First, determine that the patient is pulseless before even thinking about using the AED.
- Turn the device on as it will give both visual and auditory prompts.
- Visualize the anterior bare chest and remove any medication patches that might be on the patient's chest.
- Wipe the chest dry if wet or sweaty.
- Attach the AED pads and make sure they are connected to the device.
- Stand clear of the patient and stop CPR. Make sure everyone is clear of the patient.
- Select the analyze button and allow the device to detect the rhythm.
- If a shock is recommended, recheck to make sure everyone is clear of the patient.
- Say "stand clear" and press the "shock" button.
- After delivering the shock, begin CPR immediately and continue for two minutes before having the AED determine the rhythm again.
- If there is any spontaneous patient movement or eye opening, stop CPR and check the patient's breathing.

Key Takeaways

- AED devices have been in public use since the 1990s.
- AED devices are mandated for use in airplanes but not anywhere else.
- The AED is 100 percent specific in detecting ventricular fibrillation.
- The first step in using an AED device is to determine that the patient is pulseless.
- CPR should continue after the shock for two minutes unless there is spontaneous movement.

Quiz

1. What is the approximate survival rate of an out-of-hospital cardiac arrest when an AED is used?
   a. 10 percent
   b. 20 percent
   c. 30 percent
   d. 40 percent

Answer: c. The approximate survival rate of an out-of-hospital cardiac arrest when an AED is used is about 30 percent. The survival rate is highly dependent upon the time it takes to apply and deploy the device.

2. What is the approximate survival rate of ventricular fibrillation if only CPR is use without access to an AED?
   a. 1 percent
   b. 6 percent
   c. 10 percent
   d. 16 percent

Answer: b. About six percent of people with ventricular fibrillation survive their arrest if only CPR is used and not an AED.

3. When was it mandated that AEDs be in place on commercial airlines?
   a. 1989
   b. 1999
   c. 2001
   d. 2004

Answer: d. It was in 2004 that passenger airlines in the US were mandated to have AEDs on board with personnel trained in their use.

4. What can be said about the survival rate using an AED versus a manual defibrillator?
   a. There is no difference in survival rate.

b. The AED survival rate is slightly less than the survival rate with a manual defibrillator.

c. Because the AED is faster, the survival rate to discharge is almost twice that of a manual defibrillator.

d. AEDs used by trained professionals is superior to AEDs used by laypeople.

Answer: c. Because the AED delivers a shock faster than waiting for EMTs to use a manual defibrillator, the survival rate is almost twice as good with an AED when compared to manual defibrillation.

5. What is considered the key determining factor in having success with defibrillation in the field?
   a. Whether it is done by a layperson or first-responder
   b. The actual amount of energy produced per shock
   c. The age of the patient
   d. The time from witnessed arrest to shocking the patient

Answer: d. The key factor in survivability using an AED is the time from witnessed arrest to shocking the patient. Those patients who have an unwitnessed arrest have a low success rate, regardless of how the shock is given and who delivers the shock.

6. What is true of getting a "check electrode" message on the AED?
   a. The electrode is probably on hairy skin and needs to be put in a different spot.
   b. The electrodes are probably defective and should be replaced.
   c. The skin should be dried off more and the electrodes should be put back in the same spot.
   d. The skin should be shaved and the electrodes replaced.

Answer: b. The message "check electrode" is most commonly due to defective electrodes so they need to be replaced with a new set of electrodes.

7. AEDs are found in many areas and have been found to be successful. Where is it that AEDs are mandated to be located?
   a. In airports
   b. In health clubs
   c. On airplanes
   d. In casinos

Answer: c. The only place where AEDs are mandated to be placed is in airplanes. The other places do not have mandated placement of AEDs, although they are frequently found in these places.

8. At what age or less is it contraindicated to use an AED?
   a. Less than 18 years
   b. Less than 12 years
   c. Less than 8 years

d. Less than 1 year

Answer: d. While using an AED on a child under the age of 8 years gives a charge that is technically too much, it is better to give too much than it is to give no shock at all. The advantage shifts at one year of age or less, when it is contraindicated to use an AED under this age.

9. What is the first step to be done when deciding to use an AED?
   a. Determine that the patient is pulseless.
   b. Read the AED instruction booklet.
   c. Apply the AED electrodes.
   d. Turn on the AED machine.

Answer: a. It is important to determine that the patient is pulseless before considering applying the electrodes or turning on the device. It should not be necessary to read any manual or booklet.

10. What is the next step to do after the patient has been shocked with the AED device?
    a. Allow the AED to recheck the rhythm.
    b. Observe the patient for spontaneous movement.
    c. Perform CPR for two minutes.
    d. Recheck the pulse.

Answer: c. Regardless of the shock, CPR should be continued for two minutes before rechecking the rhythm or pulse. The only reason to not do CPR would be if the patient is spontaneously moving and breathing.

Chapter 5: Advanced Life Support Rhythm Strip Interpretation

The first part of Advanced Life Support involves recognizing the various cardiac rhythms that need to be intervened upon in patients having a cardiorespiratory problem. There is a variety of different rhythms that will be encountered by the provider of ACLS and that will ultimately lead to specific algorithms involving defibrillation, synchronous cardioversion, pacing, or medications. This chapter focuses exclusively on the various rhythms involved in the practice of ACLS.

The Rhythm Strip

In the provision of ACLS, there is the advantage over BLS in that, in the vast majority of situations, there is a rhythm strip that can guide the provider in identifying the patient's problem and in determining the next steps to take. The basic rhythm strip is different from a full ECG test in that it only involves one lead. Even so, it can identify what the basic rhythm is and can define the next few steps to be taken in caring for the patient.

The major events in a rhythm strip include the P wave, the QRS complex, the T wave, and the U wave. The first three things are found in any normal sinus rhythm, while the U wave is only found in certain circumstances. The P wave indicates the contraction of the atrium; the QRS complex indicates both depolarization and contraction of the ventricle, and is taller than the P wave.

The QRS complex is spikey, having a deflection downward (the Q component), a tall upward and downward inflection (the R component), and a deflection (the S component). After the QRS complex Is the T wave, which represents the repolarization and relaxation phase of the ventricles.

Atrial Arrhythmias

Most atrial arrhythmias are compatible with having a pulse but the pulse can be slow, normal, or rapid, depending on the patient's condition and the specific rhythm. Rhythms that involve an atrial focus tend to be faster than rhythms that have lost their atrial focus (such as atrial fibrillation) because the fastest pacemaker in the heart is in the atrium. Any rhythm that originates other than in the sinoatrial node of the left atrium tends to be slower than a rhythm that starts in the SA node.

There are several Atrial arrhythmias that are clinically significant:

- **Sinus Tachycardia.** This basically represents a normal sinus rhythm with a rate that is faster than 100 beats per minute. The pacemaker of the heart is in the sinoatrial (SA) node but has sympathetic nerve input that increases the rate. A normal sinus rhythm has a rate of between sixty and one hundred beats per minute and, when there is stress, exercise, caffeine, nicotine, or other stimulant, there is increased stimulation of the SA node so that the overall heart rate is greater than normal. The P wave, QRS complex, and T wave appear normal but just happen at a faster than normal rate. Rest and relaxation, along with decreasing stimulant activity, will improve sinus tachycardia, which otherwise needs no particular treatment.

Figure 6 indicates what sinus tachycardia looks like on ECG:

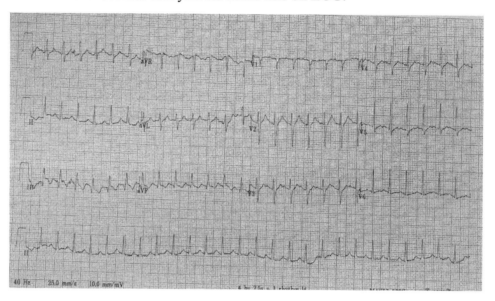

Figure 6

- **Premature Atrial Contractions.** In general, the P waves are present with a normal QRS interval and normal QRS complex. What is present is the finding of multiple early P waves, which happen before the expected time. Premature atrial beats are called PACs and can happen in normal individuals. The main causes of PACs include excess stress, exercising too much, having too much caffeine, or taking in too much nicotine. They are not considered serious and are generally not treated, although relaxation and deep breathing can decrease the number of PACs. The pacemaker of the heart in PACs is still the normal sinoatrial node but the node is stimulated to do "extra" beats that slightly increase the heart rate and make it slightly irregular.
- **Atrial flutter.** This involves a rhythm that originates in the sinoatrial node but the rate is much faster than a normal sinus rhythm. There can be 1:1 conduction of the atrial beat, 2:1 conduction of the atrial beat, 3:1 conduction of the atrial beat, or lesser degrees of conduction, although this would be less common. The P wave is abnormally shaped and forms a "saw-tooth pattern" that has the maximal sinoatrial rate of about three

hundred impulses per minute. Very rarely would this be possible at a 1:1 conduction rate. At this rate, the ventricles would not have enough time to relax between contractions and the cardiac output would be severely diminished. More commonly is 2:1 conduction, with a ventricular rate of 150. The rhythm is considered a re-entrant rhythm involving either the left or right atrium. It starts in a premature atrial beat that travels through the atria and gets propagated over and over again in a self-perpetuating loop. The atrioventricular node or AV node is protective and prevents 1:1 conduction so that the ventricular rate is a half or less than the atrial rate. The block can be enhanced so the rate is slowed even further. In later chapters, we will talk about the medications that can slow the rate in this arrhythmia.

Figure 7 shows atrial flutter on ECG:

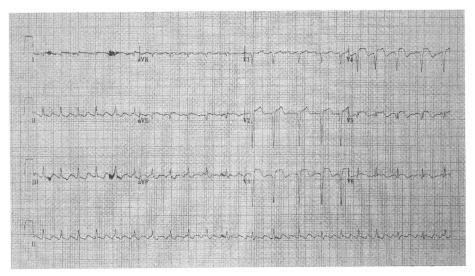

Figure 7

- **Atrial Fibrillation.** Atrial fibrillation (AF) is a common abnormal heart rhythm. The rate tends to be fast and there is irregular or no beating of the atria. It can start with atrial flutter and degenerate from there. Patients may have chest pain and palpitations because of the rapid rate, lightheadedness, palpitations, and fainting spells. The main risk factors for atrial fibrillation are valvular heart disease and high blood pressure, although congenital heart disease, cardiomyopathy, coronary artery disease, and heart failure can cause atrial fibrillation. Patients with thyrotoxicosis, diabetes mellitus, excessive alcohol intake, obesity, sleep apnea, and COPD will have a non-cardiac risk factor for atrial fibrillation. The rhythm strip is characteristic because there is a complete absence of a P wave with a fibrillating baseline. The QRS complex and T wave are generally normal in appearance and the rhythm is almost always irregular. This represents the most commonly seen serious arrhythmia, with a prevalence rate of about 2-3 percent of the total adult population in the US. One of the big problems with AF is that blood can collect in the atria, causing a clot that can break off, leading to an embolic stroke. Patients with this problem need blood thinners to prevent a stroke. Some patients can have heart failure because they need the atrial "kick" to have a good cardiac output.

- **Sinus Bradycardia.** This is a rhythm that originates in the sinoatrial node and may be normal in athletes (who tend to have a slower heart rate). The rate is, by definition, less than 60 beats per minute with an otherwise normal P wave, QRS complex, and T wave. Pathological causes of sinus bradycardia include sick sinus syndrome and medications which slow the heart rate (digoxin, beta-blockers, calcium channel-blockers). There are many other drugs unrelated to the heart directly that can cause sinus bradycardia, but this is less common. Sleep apnea, hypoglycemia, and hypothermia can cause sinus bradycardia.

Figure 8 shows sinus bradycardia with a sinus pause:

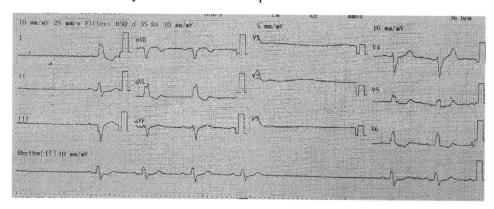

Figure 8

Junctional Rhythms

There are several junctional rhythms that determine the heart rate and rhythm. In such cases, the origin of the heartbeat is in the atrioventricular node (AV node) rather than the SA node.

- **Junctional rhythm.** This arrhythmia can happen when there is an impulse from the atrium that is slower than the rate that can be supplied by the AV node. This is an escape rhythm that has a rate of 40-60 beats per minute. There is usually a normal, narrow QRS complex with or without a retrograde P wave. An accelerated junctional rhythm with a rate greater than sixty bpm can be seen in things like recent heart surgery, acute coronary syndrome, isoproterenol infusion, and digitalis toxicity.
- **Junctional Ectopic Tachycardia.** This is an arrhythmia which has a rapid heart rate driven by the AV node of the heart. The QRS complex is normal in appearance and there are usually retrograde P waves seen at the end of the QRS complex. There are two types of this rhythm disturbance. The first is idiopathic junctional ectopic

tachycardia, which usually has a structurally normal heart. The second is "transient postoperative junctional ectopic tachycardia", which is seen after surgery for congenital heart disease. The incidence of this rhythm after heart surgery is about 14 percent; it is secondary to handling of the heart and inflammation of the conductive tissue after surgery. It is the most common cause of this type of rhythm and it tends to abate spontaneously after 36 hours. Idiopathic disease that is congenital is hard to treat and often requires ablation, pacemaker insertion, and/or multiple antiarrhythmic drugs. Digoxin toxicity can show junctional toxicity that is not paroxysmal in nature.

- **Supraventricular Tachycardia.** This is a rapid rhythm that is fast enough to be symptomatic, with palpitations, lightheadedness, and fainting. It is characterized by a sudden onset and termination of a rapid, narrow QRS rhythm. It is initiated in the AV node and has a regular rhythm. It can occur in all ages and can be hard to treat. This is a reentry rhythm in which the beat comes cyclically. There are premature ventricular ectopic beats that repeat at a rate greater than 100 and generally at a rate that is about 150-160 bpm. Triggers include being hyperthyroid and substances, such as alcohol, drugs, and caffeine. It can be seen in digoxin toxicity and in many types of heart disease, including having a previous myocardial infarction, pericarditis, and rheumatic heart disease.

Figure 9 demonstrates supraventricular tachycardia:

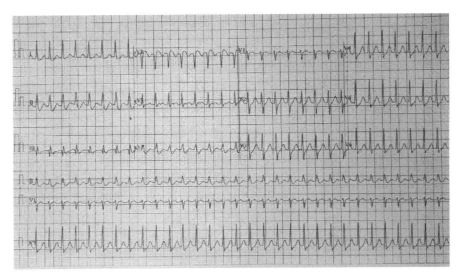

Figure 9

Ventricular Rhythms

These tend to be more severe rhythms with a greater chance of pathology in the heart, more symptoms, and a greater chance of death [except for PVCs (premature ventricular contractions)].

- **Premature ventricular contractions (PVCs).** These are caused by an ectopic heart pacemaker located somewhere in the ventricle. The actual QRS complex seen in a PVC is highly abnormal and wide-complex in nature. They are not preceded by any P wave and have an oppositely-deflected, large T wave. It can be secondary to a reentry beat, an area of enhanced automaticity, or a trigger to a part of the ventricle. Enhanced automaticity and PVCs can be seen in electrolyte problems (especially hypokalemia) or excesses of catecholamines. The ECG pattern will show a large R wave and a left bundle branch block. The main treatment for this is beta-blocker medications. PVCs can be due to heart problems, such as an acute MI, myocardial contusion, cardiomyopathy, myocarditis, or mitral valve prolapse. Non-cardiac causes of PVCs include hypercapnia, hypoxia, stimulant illicit substances, tobacco use, alcohol use, tricyclic antidepressants, digoxin, and aminophylline. Electrolyte imbalances likely to lead to PVCs include hypercalcemia, hypokalemia, and hypomagnesemia.

- **Ventricular Tachycardia.** Ventricular tachycardia is one of the top causes of sudden death in the US, along with ventricular fibrillation. Ventricular tachycardia involves a rhythm of faster than 100 beats per minute that has at least three beats in a row that is generated by the ventricles instead of the atria. It can come from the ventricular conducting system or the myocardium itself. The rate can be as fast as 300 beats per minute with dissociated P wave absent or present (buried beneath the wide-complex QRS). When the ventricular tachycardia is between 240 and 300 bpm, it is called ventricular flutter. At this rate, the patient may not be able to perfuse their brain so they may be lightheaded, feel faint, be hypotensive, and will have a high jugular venous pressure because the cardiac output is poor. The ECG strip will show a run of at least three wide QRS complexes that are relatively regular and will occur at an extremely rapid rate. Things that precipitate ventricular tachycardia include digoxin toxicity, hypocalcemia, hypokalemia, and hypomagnesemia. Recreational drug use can cause it as can a myocardial injury (such as a myocardial infarction.

Figure 10 indicates a rhythm strip with ventricular tachycardia:

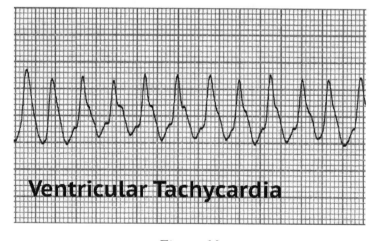

Figure 10

- **Ventricular Fibrillation.** Ventricular fibrillation is the most life-threatening of all arrhythmias except for possibly asystole (which is not technically an arrhythmia because it represents an absence of any cardiac electrical activity). In cardiac arrest patients, this rhythm represents up to 85 percent of all rhythms detected by EMS services. The use of the AED in the field has increased the survivability of this otherwise very serious rhythm disturbance. The ECG can show fine or coarse irregular electrical activity with no definable P waves, QRS complex, or T waves. Patents who are prone to this rhythm can have an implantable cardioverter-defibrillator (ICD), which can defibrillate as soon as the rhythm presents itself. It is highly linked to coronary artery disease and the presence of an acute myocardial infarction or from scar tissue around an old myocardial infarction. It can come on suddenly but often represents a degeneration of ventricular tachycardia. Among survivors of ventricular fibrillation, about 85 percent will have some type of coronary artery blockage—most often more than one vessel. About 10 percent of ventricular fibrillation cases will have a cardiomyopathy without ischemia (dilated cardiomyopathy, hypertrophic cardiomyopathy, or other type of rarer cardiomyopathy).

Figure 11 shows coarse ventricular fibrillation:

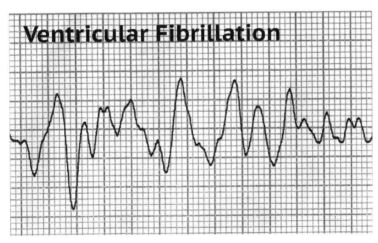

Figure 11

- **Torsade de pointes.** This is a relatively uncommon type of ventricular tachycardia in which the QRS complexes are wide and differ in appearance from one another—appearing to twist around the isoelectric line. It is highly linked to long QT syndrome, which can be congenital or acquired. It often goes away on its own but can degenerate into ventricular fibrillation, similar to uncomplicated ventricular tachycardia. The QT interval is markedly prolonged, which is another way to differentiate it from regular ventricular tachycardia. There are two rare congenital syndromes associated with long QT syndrome, including Lange-Nielsen syndrome and Jervell syndrome—both of which are complicated by sudden death secondary to ventricular fibrillation or Torsade de pointes that degenerates into VF. Electrolyte disturbances most closely linked to acquired torsade include hypomagnesemia and hypokalemia. Drugs most closely linked to getting Torsades de pointes include Class IC anti-arrhythmics, certain antihistamine drugs, phenothiazines, lithium, tricyclic antidepressants, cisapride, antiretroviral drugs, ziprasidone, and some chemotherapy drugs. Torsades de pointes can be associated with various endocrine disorders, myocardial infarction, intracranial disorders, and nutritional problems (such as anorexia, celiac disease, and starvation).

Figure 12 shows a typical rhythm strip with this arrythmia:

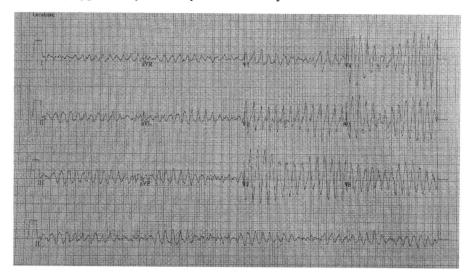

Figure 12

Heart Block Rhythms

Some rhythm disturbances are secondary to some degree of heart block. Heart block can range from first degree heart block (which has very few symptoms) to third degree heart block (which can be very symptomatic). Second degree heart block can be type 1 (Mobitz I), which is a relatively benign disease or type 2 (Mobitz II), which carries more ominous implications.

- **First Degree Heart Block.** First degree atrioventricular (AV) block or simply first-degree heart block is basically a prolonged PR interval that is longer than 200 milliseconds in duration. The PR interval begins at the start of the P wave and ends at the beginning of the QRS complex. The conduction is slower than expected but no beats are missed so both the atrial and ventricular rate are regular and the same. The delay in function is usually secondary to some type of pathology of the AV node, which normally takes the atrial impulse and transmits an impulse that makes the QRS complex in the ventricles. A first-degree heart block can also be secondary to an inferior wall myocardial infarction, hypomagnesemia, hypokalemia, athletic training (because of increased vagal tone), antiarrhythmic medications, calcification of the mitral or aortic valve, infective endocarditis, collagen vascular disease, or having an adenosine stress test.

- **Second Degree Heart Block.** There are two types of second-degree heart block. In second-degree heart block, there is a delay in conduction of the impulse through the AV node with skipping of some of the beats. Patients may have no symptoms or may have symptoms of low blood pressure, chest pain, heart rate irregularity, bradycardia, or syncope. Type 1 (Mobitz I or Wenckebach AV block) is the most common type of second-degree block. In this condition, there is progressive prolongation of the PR interval until a ventricular beat is missed. This happens every few beats, resulting in a dropped beat that may be symptomatic. This is considered to be a more benign form of second-degree heart block when compared to Mobitz II second-degree heart block. In this form of heart block, the patient has several normal beats followed by a missed beat. The ventricular rate is about half that or a third that of the atrial rate. For example, in 2:1 second-degree AV block, the P wave is picked up and associated with a QRS complex every other P wave, making the atrial rate twice that of the ventricular rate. This is much more likely to degenerate into a third-degree AV block when compared to a Mobitz I second-degree AV block.

Figure 13 shows Mobitz I heart block:

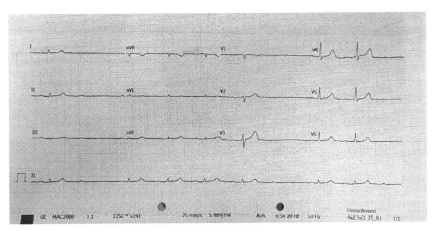

Figure 13

- **Third Degree Heart Block.** Third-degree heart block is also called complete heart block because there is no association between the P wave and the QRS complex. The P wave has its own rate and the ventricular escape rhythm kicks in to have a separate ventricular rate and a dissociated QRS complex. The QRS can originate anywhere from the AV node to the Purkinje system in the ventricular wall. Anything that disrupts the electrical conduction system, such as fibrosis, infiltration, or infarction of the electrical tissue can adversely affect the connection between the atria and ventricles. Patients often present with severe bradycardia. Often, the only treatment is to pace the patient's ventricular rhythm so that it is fast enough to bring up the cardiac output. When the escape rhythm comes from the AV node, the ventricular rate is about 45-60 beats per minute which may or may not be symptomatic. If the escape rhythm comes from the bundle-branch Purkinje system of the ventricles (distal to the AV node), the heart rate is about 45 beats per minute or less. These patients are generally quite symptomatic.

Figure 14 demonstrates third degree heart block:

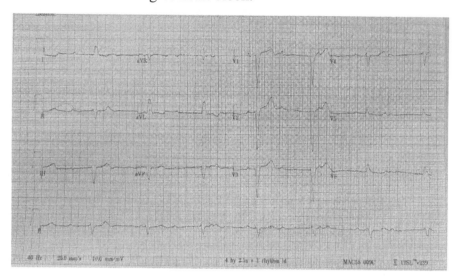

Figure 14

Key Takeaways

- The ECG rhythm strip is the best way to determine the patient's status as it indicates the electrical activity of the heart.
- There are atrial arrhythmias. Ventricular arrhythmias, and heart blocks that can be symptomatic and that will activate the various ACLS protocols.
- In general, ventricular arrhythmias are considered more life-threatening than atrial arrhythmias.
- Heart block rhythms involve a delay in transmission or dissociation of the atrial and ventricular electrical impulses.

Quiz

1. What part of a normal sinus rhythm (NSR) strip is not seen in all cases of NSR?
   a. P wave
   b. QRS complex
   c. T wave
   d. U wave

Answer: d. The U wave isn't seen in all cases of a normal sinus rhythm but is seen in select cases. The other elements must be present for the rhythm to be considered NSR.

2. Which part of the normal sinus rhythm represents the time that the ventricles are contracting?
   a. P wave
   b. QRS complex
   c. T wave
   d. U wave

Answer: b. The QRS complex represents the time when the ventricles are contracting.

3. What technique or drug can reduce the number of PACs the patient has?
   a. Deep breathing and relaxation
   b. Caffeine
   c. Nicotine
   d. Excessive exercise

Answer: a. Deep breathing and relaxation can effectively reduce the number of PVCs the patient has. The other choices will increase the number of PVCs the patient has.

4. Which is not considered a non-cardiac risk factor for atrial fibrillation?
   a. COPD
   b. Thyrotoxicosis
   c. Coronary artery disease
   d. Sleep apnea

Answer: c. There are many non-cardiac causes of atrial fibrillation, including obesity, sleep apnea, diabetes mellitus, thyrotoxicosis, and COPD. Coronary artery disease will be a cardiac risk factor for atrial fibrillation.

5. What will the characteristics be of the P wave in atrial fibrillation?
   a. It is peaked.
   b. It is prolonged.
   c. It is shorter than normal.
   d. It does not exist.

Answer: d. The P wave does not exist in atrial fibrillation, which is characteristic of atrial fibrillation.

6. What is considered to be the most common serious arrhythmia that can be found in the US adult population?
   a. Atrial flutter
   b. Atrial fibrillation
   c. Supraventricular tachycardia
   d. Sinus bradycardia

Answer: b. Atrial fibrillation is an extremely common arrhythmia, affecting 2-4 percent of the adult population, with the prevalence increasing with age.

7. Which is not considered a cause of an accelerated junctional rhythm?
    a. Digitalis toxicity
    b. Acute coronary syndrome
    c. Recent heart surgery
    d. Atropine infusion

Answer: d. All of the above can cause an accelerated junctional rhythm except for atropine infusion.

8. What is considered to be a main cause of junctional escape tachycardia?
    a. Surgery on the heart
    b. Beta-blocker toxicity
    c. Idiopathic congenital junctional escape tachycardia
    d. Anti-arrhythmic toxicity

Answer: a. A common cause of junctional escape tachycardia is surgery on the heart. Manipulation of the heart and inflammation of the conduction tissue is believed to cause this type of transient rhythm, which usually resolves within 36 hours of surgery.

9. Which cardiac arrhythmia leads most to the chance of having an embolic stroke?
    a. Atrial flutter
    b. Atrial fibrillation
    c. Sinus bradycardia
    d. Supraventricular tachycardia

Answer: b. Patients with atrial fibrillation have a higher than normal risk of an embolic stroke because the blood pools in the atria and causes clots to form that can break off and go to the brain.

10. If a patient has a complete heart block and the ventricular escape rhythm comes from the bundle-branch Purkinje system, what is the ventricular rate?
    a. Less than 45 bpm
    b. 45-60 bpm
    c. 55-80 bpm
    d. Greater than 100 bpm

Answer: a. If the ventricular escape rhythm comes below the level of the AV node, such as in the bundle-branch Purkinje system, the ventricular rate would be less than 45 beats per minute.

Chapter 6: Arrhythmia Algorithms

This chapter of the course continues with discussions related to Advanced Cardiac Life Support. In chapter 5, the focus of the discussion was on the arrhythmias a provide might come in contact with as part of ACLS practice. This chapter now focuses on the algorithms the ACLS provider uses in order to evaluate and treat patients who have the various rhythm disturbances, with a special focus on those arrhythmias that are symptomatic and result in a patient with a relatively unstable clinical situation. Each type of rhythm disturbance is treated with a different algorithm. The focus of this chapter is on the algorithms as a whole with a discussion in a later chapter on the medications used in these algorithms.

ACLS Tachycardia Algorithm for Stable Tachycardia

The crucial thing to decide in a patient with tachycardia of any etiology is to see if they have a pulse. This can identify whether or not the patient is stable and will define the treatment used. If the patient doesn't have a pulse, the ACLS Pulseless Arrest Algorithm will be followed. If the patient has a pulse, the ACLS Tachycardia Algorithm should be followed.

A stable tachycardia depends on a heart rate greater than a hundred beats per minute and no evidence of hypoxia or other serious symptoms associated with having a fast rhythm. After assessing the pulse, ask the patient how they are feeling in order to determine if they are symptomatic. If the patient has a pulse but is highly symptomatic with lightheadedness shortness of breath, faintness, or extreme palpitations, they need immediate cardioversion with a synchronized cardioversion.

Do a rhythm strip. Check to see if the QRS complex is narrow or wide and check to see if the rhythm is regular or irregular. If the patient is having sinus tachycardia, they need to relax and take deep breaths. Sinus tachycardia is the only stable tachycardia that does not need any treatment and does not need cardioversion as relaxation can bring the rate down.

If the patient is pulseless and has ventricular tachycardia, the pulseless arrest algorithm is indicated and an unsynchronized high energy shock (or several shocks) needs to be given immediately. If the patient has polymorphic ventricular tachycardia an is unstable, the rhythm should be treated the same as ventricular fibrillation (even if a pulse is present and the patient is hypotensive). Unsynchronized high energy shocks should be given.

If the patient has a stable tachycardia, check the airway, breathing, and circulation. Provide oxygen by mask and check an O2 saturation. Get a 12-lead ECG to see what the rhythm is and check the blood pressure. Identify the rhythm and treat any reversible causes of stable tachycardia. Look for evidence of altered mental status, hypotension, shock, or continued chest pain, which would indicate possible instability. If the rate is less than 150 bpm, the patient is unlikely to be unstable or have severe symptoms. Start an IV on all stable patients and follow their rhythm strip.

Check to see if the QRS is narrow or wide. If the QRS is narrow and the rhythm is regular, the patient may have SVT. Try vagal maneuvers first and then give adenosine at six milligrams IV push. If this fails to convert the patient, two additional doses of twelve milligrams IV push of adenosine should be given. Supraventricular tachycardia will usually convert with adenosine. If it recurs, longer-acting agents like beta-blockers or diltiazem can be given, which are longer-acting atrioventricular nodal blockers.

If the patient has a narrow QRS rhythm strip but an irregular rate, the three choices for a diagnosis are atrial flutter, wandering atrial pacemaker tachycardia, or atrial fibrillation. The treatment for symptoms is to control the heart rate with beta-blockers or diltiazem. Beta-blockers need to be use with caution in asthma, other lung diseases, and congestive heart failure.

If the patient has a wide QRS complex (greater than 0.12 seconds) and a regular rhythm, the patient should be treated with amiodarone 150 mg IV over ten minutes and this can be repeated to control the rate until as much as 2.2 grams of the drug are given over twenty-four hours. The patient needs to be sedated in preparation for elective synchronized cardioversion. This is likely a stable ventricular tachycardia.

If the patient has atrial fibrillation and known Wolff-Parkinson-White syndrome, AV nodal blocking agents will make the condition worse so things like adenosine, digoxin, verapamil, and diltiazem. If the patient has an obvious Torsades de pointes tachycardia, the treatment is magnesium (1-2 grams IV over 5-20 minutes, flowed by an infusion).

At any time the patient becomes unstable, treat immediately with something like synchronized or unsynchronized cardioversion without taking the time to analyze the rhythm as the treatment with cardioversion is the same regardless of the actual rhythm the patient is exhibiting.

Pulseless Algorithm secondary to Asystole or PEA

PEA stands for "pulseless electrical activity", which is treated identically to asystole. The goal is to identify any underlying, treatable problem and treat it rather than just treating the rhythm. Asystole, if present, should be documented in two leads in order to prove the diagnosis.

The first step is to check the rhythm in two leads to verify asystole. Start CPR at 100-120 beats per minute, with respirations/ventilations per CPR protocol. Start an IV as soon as one is available and give 1 mg epinephrine IV while CPR is ongoing. Intubate as soon as possible.

Consider the possible causes:

- Hypothermia
- Drug overdose
- Preexisting acidosis
- Hypokalemia
- Hyperkalemia

- Hypoxia

After giving the epinephrine and doing CPR to circulate it for two minutes, check the rhythm. If there is electrical activity on the rhythm strip, check the pulse. If there is no pulse, CPR should be continued and epinephrine repeated e very three to five minutes. IV access and epinephrine injection should take precedence over establishing an airway. After doing this several times, it is up to the team to decide when to terminate resuscitative efforts as asystole has a very poor prognosis.

Algorithm for Ventricular Fibrillation (VF) and Pulseless Ventricular Tachycardia (VT)

When facing an unconscious patient without a pulse, start basic BLS protocol and determine if the patient has a pulse and that they are unconscious. Activate the EMS system and call for a defibrillator while CPR is started.

The first treatment of choice once ventricular fibrillation is documented or suspected is to defibrillate up to three times over several minutes. If the VT/VF is persistent, give epinephrine, 1 mg IV push, repeated every three to five minutes, while CPR is given. Other medications that might help but are given secondarily include lidocaine, bretyllium, magnesium sulfate, and procainamide. Sodium bicarbonate is a third-line agent given if acidosis is strongly suspected. Shocking should be done between giving doses of medication.

The ACLS Bradycardia Algorithm

The first thing to do is to determine that the patient has a pulse and that the pulse is less than 60 beats per minute. This identifies bradycardia. Make sure the airway is intact and start oxygen if the O2 sat is 94 percent or less (or if the patient is dyspneic). Obtain access with an IV and look for treatable causes of the problem.

Determine if the patient has symptoms or signs of underperfusion. Do they have increased chest congestion suggestive of pulmonary edema, altered mental status, weakness, dyspnea, chest pain, lightheadedness, hypotension, or syncope and are these symptoms connected to the bradycardia? Monitor the patient if they are perfusing and treat with oxygen, IV access, and observation.

If the patient is not perfusing, get a rhythm strip. If the patient has heart block, consider transcutaneous pacing, which should be done even before an IV access has been obtained. Pacing is the first-line treatment, but, if this is not available, start atropine 0.5 mg IV every three to five minutes for up to six doses.

Only if pacing and atropine are found to be ineffective, consider IV epinephrine, dopamine, or isoproterenol. These can be given while waiting for a pacemaker and may bring the rate up at least temporarily. The dose of epinephrine is 2-10 micrograms per minute infusion. The dose of dopamine is an infusion of 2-10 micrograms per kilogram per minute.

ACLS Algorithm for Unstable Tachycardia

The first goal is to determine that the patient is tachycardic and the second goal is to recognize whether or not the patient is stable. If the pulse is between 100 and 150, the problem is likely something secondary to sinus tachycardia. Rates higher than this will likely be symptomatic. Patients with underlying heart disease will have symptoms at rates lower than 150 beats per minute. If the rate is over 150 and the patient is symptomatic, the treatment of choice will be synchronized cardioversion. If sinus tachycardia is suspected, treatment of the underlying cause is the mainstay of treatment.

First, determine if the patient has a pulse. If they have a pulse, do a 12-lead EKG and give O2 if the patient has an O2 sat of less than 94 percent or if they complain of shortness of breath. Identify the rhythm and check a blood pressure. If stable, look for underlying causes and treat. If cardioversion is planned and the patient is not unconscious, give them sedation to prevent the pain and agitation that will occur with cardioversion.

If the QRS complex is narrow, try vagal maneuvers first and then follow with a 6-mg adenosine IV push. If this is unsuccessful, repeat with a 12-mg adenosine IV push. If the patient converts, the tachycardia was atrial in origin.

If the patient has a narrow complex QRS complex and an irregular rhythm, the rate should be controlled with either diltiazem or beta-blockers. An irregular, narrow complex rhythm is likely to be atrial flutter or atrial fibrillation and these rhythms can be rate-controlled.

Wide QRS complexes suggest a ventricular rhythm, such as ventricular tachycardia. If IV access has been obtained, give amiodarone 150 mg IV over ten minutes, repeated up to 2.2 grams total. Cardiovert if the patient is unstable. Amiodarone should be given for atrial fibrillation in the setting of Wolff-Parkinson White syndrome and adenosine should be avoided. Any time there is a wide QRS complex rhythm, you need to assume ventricular tachycardia until proven otherwise.

Algorithm for Pulmonary Edema

The patient with pulmonary edema represents a complicated problem. They have either volume depletion, a pump problem, or a heart rate problem (with either a fast or slow rhythm). The treatment of volume depleted pulmonary edema and shock includes giving an IV bolus of fluid, which should restore the volume status of the patient. If the systolic blood pressure (BP) is low, start norepinephrine IV. If this doesn't work, try giving dopamine.

If the patient has a pump problem, pulmonary edema, and a normal blood pressure, the initial treatment of choice is dopamine (if symptomatic with shock) or dobutamine (if no evidence of shock). If the patient has a pump problem and has an elevated blood pressure, the treatment of choice for the first-line agent is nitroglycerin IV, followed by nitroprusside, which will decrease the blood pressure and improve pump function.

All patients with pulmonary edema should have morphine, IV furosemide, sublingual nitroglycerin, and oxygen, intubating them if they have problems with spontaneous respirations. Third-line agents include amrinone, aminophylline (if wheezing), and digoxin (to enhance pump activity and improve cardiac output). The goal is to improve pumping activity of the heart, draw fluid out of the lungs, maintain oxygenation, and treat any underlying cause for the pulmonary edema.

Key Takeaways

- There are various protocols and algorithms to follow that are based on what the patient's heart rate is, the width of the QRS complex, and the patient's cardiorespiratory status.
- Wide-complex QRS rhythms should be considered to be ventricular tachycardia until proven otherwise.
- The rhythm problem is considered to be atrial in origin if adenosine IV push resolves the tachycardia immediately.
- The first-line treatment for any bradycardic rhythm is transcutaneous pacemaker placement.

Quiz

1. When treating the patient with tachycardia, what is the first thing that needs to be determined in order to decide the algorithm to use?
   a. The patient's pulse oximetry reading
   b. A 12-lead EKG determination
   c. Whether or not the patient has a pulse
   d. A relatively exact determination of the pulse rate

Answer: c. The choice of algorithm and the actual first determination in tachycardic patients is to see if they have a pulse. The algorithm is different if they have a pulse versus not having a pulse.

2. Which type of tachycardia requires no real treatment?
   a. Sinus tachycardia
   b. Supraventricular tachycardia
   c. Atrial flutter
   d. Atrial fibrillation with rapid ventricular response

Answer: a. Regardless of symptoms, no treatment is necessary for sinus tachycardia except for relaxing and taking deep breaths.

3. You have successfully treated a patient with supraventricular tachycardia using rapidly-acting adenosine but the rhythm returns. The patient is symptomatic with palpitations but is otherwise stable. What can be given?
   a. Atropine
   b. Diltiazem
   c. Guanfecine
   d. Amiodarone

Answer: b. The treatment of choice for recurrent SVT is to give a longer-acting AV nodal reentry blocker, such as diltiazem or a beta-blocker.

4. What is the initial drug of choice in treating a patient with asystole?
   a. Atropine IV
   b. Adenosine IV
   c. Epinephrine IV
   d. Amiodarone IV

Answer: c. The only real treatment for asystole besides treating the underlying causes and CPR is epinephrine given while CPR is ongoing every 3-5 minutes.

5. In managing a patient with ventricular fibrillation who is unconscious and has no pulse, what is the treatment of choice for initial care?
   a. Defibrillate up to three times
   b. Epinephrine IV
   c. Sodium bicarbonate IV
   d. Atropine IV

Answer: a. Ventricular fibrillation is best managed with repeated attempts at defibrillating the patient. Epinephrine is used if this does not successfully defibrillate the patient.

6. In managing the patient with symptomatic bradycardia and hypoperfusion, what is the first-line treatment?
   a. Atropine IV
   b. Transcutaneous pacing
   c. Epinephrine IV
   d. Dopamine infusion

Answer: b. The first line treatment of bradycardia that is symptomatic, regardless of the rhythm, is to begin transcutaneous pacing, which can be done even before the IV access has been obtained.

7. What can you give a tachycardic patient to prove that their tachycardia was atrial in origin?
   a. IV propranolol
   b. IV digoxin

c. IV adenosine

d. IV amiodarone

Answer: c. If you give the patient with tachycardia IV adenosine and they convert, you can prove that the patient has an atrial tachycardia. This is diagnostic of the atrial origin to the arrhythmia.

8. When treating a wide QRS complex tachycardia with an IV access, what is the drug treatment of choice as a first-line agent?
   a. Amiodarone
   b. Magnesium sulfate
   c. Epinephrine
   d. Propranolol

Answer: a. If an IV access has been established and the rhythm has a wide QRS complex, treat the patient with IV amiodarone as a first-line agent, which can convert a ventricular tachycardia to NSR.

9. The patient is unstable and has a rhythm strip showing a wide QRS complex form. What rhythm should be assumed with this?
   a. Atrial fibrillation with Wolff-Parkinson-White syndrome
   b. Ventricular tachycardia
   c. Torsades de pointes
   d. Pulseless electrical activity

Answer: b. Any time the QRS is wide, ventricular tachycardia should be assumed unless it is proven otherwise be an expert cardiologist.

10. What is not considered a first-line agent for a patient with pulmonary edema?
    a. Furosemide
    b. Sublingual nitroglycerin
    c. Theophylline
    d. IV morphine

Answer: c. All of the above treatments are appropriate first-line treatments for pulmonary edema except for theophylline, which is only given if the patient is wheezing and is considered a third-line treatment.

Chapter 7: ACLS Medications

So far, the course has eluded to the use of a variety of medications given to treat patients with shock, pulmonary edema, asystole, or a rhythm disturbance of the heart. Some of the discussion has covered the doses and indications for these drugs. In this chapter, we will cover the medications in more detail, including their uses, doses, and any precautions that need to be taken when using these medications in an Advanced Cardiac Life Support setting.

Medication List

The following is an exhaustive list of the various medications given in a cardiac arrest situation. Some are widely used in many arrest situations, while others are used in certain specific settings and then only under the guidance of a cardiologist or hospitalist, who are usually more familiar with giving these medications than the average ACLS provider.

Oxygen

The provision of oxygen of some sort is recommended in nearly all ACLS condition. Oxygen is generally mandatory in cases where the oxygen saturation is 94 percent or less (or if the patient complains of shortness of breath. Oxygen can be given by mask, nasal cannula or directly into an endotracheal tube. In general, 100 percent oxygen is recommended unless the patient is breathing on their own and has a history of chronic obstructive pulmonary disease (in which they stop breathing when their oxygen saturation is high as their drive to breathe stems from their degree of hypoxia). COPD patients will do best with a Venturi mask, which controls the amount of oxygen delivered.

Adenosine

Adenosine is a purine nucleoside that is known to slow conduction through the AV node. It can be used to treat patients with paroxysmal supraventricular tachycardia, supraventricular tachycardia associated with Wolff-Parkinson-White syndrome, and some cases of widened QRS tachycardia. It is one of the few drugs that must be given as a fast push. The first dose is always 6 mg IV given as quickly as possible. After observing the effect, the second dose is always 12 mg IV push. A flush must be given after that to make sure it gets into the veins and is circulated.

Side effects are common but, because it doesn't last long in the system, the side effects are brief. It must be used cautiously in asthmatics because it can cause bronchospasm. Other side effects include transient flushing, brief chest pain, sinus bradycardia, ventricular ectopy, or worsened AV block in patients with a preexisting AV block. There are rarely any long-lasting hemodynamic effects because it is given so quickly and goes away very quickly.

Amiodarone

This is an antiarrhythmic drug used to treat pulseless ventricular tachycardia, ventricular fibrillation, unstable ventricular tachycardia, and some supraventricular tachycardias. The dose is 300 mg IV push for V-tach and V-fib, while for unstable V-tach, it is given at a dose of 150 mg IV over ten minutes, followed by an infusion of 1 mg/min IV for six hours and 0.5 mg/min IV for an additional eighteen hours.

The main risks of giving amiodarone include hypotension when given as a rapid bolus. It can also cause hypotension if the total daily dose is greater than 2.2 grams per twenty-four-hour period of time. It cannot be given with a drug that might prolong the QT interval and the QT interval must be monitored while the patient is on the drug.

Atropine

Atropine is a parasympatholytic drug that increases the automaticity and conductivity of the atrioventricular node. It is primarily used in symptomatic bradycardia but can be used in asystole in situations of a cardiac arrest. It can completely resolve first-degree AV block and second-degree Mobitz I block. It can paradoxically cause a slowing of the heart rate in patients with Mobitz II and third-degree AV block so this must be monitored for.

The dose of atropine in ACLS situations is 0.5 mg to 1 mg IV every three to five minutes for a maximum total dosage of three milligrams. Giving a dose that is too little is likely to cause paradoxical bradycardia in certain patients. In rare cases, a low dose of atropine can precipitate ventricular fibrillation. It can also result in tachycardia, even when given in normal doses. Anticholinergic syndrome has been reported, which includes ataxia, blurry vision, delirium, flushed skin, and coma.

Dopamine

Dopamine is a precursor molecule to norepinephrine. It stimulates the beta-adrenergic, alpha-adrenergic, and dopaminergic receptors. Low doses produce vasodilation of the renal arteries, mesenteric arteries, and cerebral arteries. In higher doses, it stimulates the beta- and alpha-adrenergic receptors, increasing the cardiac output. High doses cause a predominant alpha-adrenergic effect.

It is given for any arrhythmia or clinical situation in which hypotension exists, except it is not indicated in hypovolemia. It can improve the outcome of bradycardia. It is especially helpful in hypotension resulting in oliguria as it improves renal blood flow. It can be given in doses as low as 1-2 micrograms per kilogram per minute in an infusion, titrated to the lowest effective dose that improves the patient's hemodynamic status. It is best given with nitroprusside in cases of increased pulmonary congestion. One big risk of infusion is extravasation of the medication in the tissues and tissue necrosis. The patient needs to be euvolemic before it can be given.

Epinephrine

Epinephrine is a natural catecholamine used for cardiac arrest situations, anaphylaxis, severe hypotension, and symptomatic bradycardia. It causes a number of effects, including increasing systemic vascular resistance, increasing blood pressure, increasing myocardial electrical activity, increased cerebral and coronary blood flow, increased myocardial contractions, increased myocardial oxygen demands, and increased automaticity.

The dose of epinephrine is almost always given intravenously, although it can be placed into the endotracheal tube. A total of 10 ml of a 1: 10,000 solution or one milligram is given every three to five minutes. An IV flush should happen after giving the drug and CPR should continue to allow the epinephrine to flow through the body. It allows for a favorable distribution of blood between the peripheral vascular and the cerebral vasculature. Because it increases blood pressure and pulse, it is a good drug to use for hypotension and shock.

In cases of arrest secondary to a beta-blocker or calcium channel blocker overdose, higher doses of the drug are necessary. After given as a bolus, a continuous infusion may be necessary. Extremely high doses don't improve neurological outcome, although some studies show improved survival after cardiac arrest in patients who received high-dose epinephrine. It can be used as an infusion in cases of shock or in the post-resuscitation period.

Lidocaine

Lidocaine is successful in cases of ventricular tachycardia and ventricular fibrillation because it suppresses ventricular arrhythmias and decreases automaticity. It can affect the conduction through the reentrant pathways causing the arrhythmia. It is used as a first-line agent but Is used for cases refractory to epinephrine. It can be used in Torsades de pointes and in polymorphic ventricular tachycardia.

The dose in a cardiac arrest situation is 1.5 mg/kg IV push, while the dose in refractory ventricular fibrillation is 0.5-0.75 mg/kg IV push given every five to ten minutes for a maximum of three doses or about three milligrams per kilogram total. In stable ventricular tachycardia, the dose is 0.5-0.75 mg/kg, given up to 1.5 mg/kg. The maximum dose is always three milligrams per kilogram. A maintenance infusion can be given at 1-4 mg/minute if it is initially successful.

The biggest precautions in giving lidocaine include that it isn't routinely recommended after a cardiac arrest unless it has been shown to be successful in resolving the rhythm problem. It shouldn't be used prophylactically after a myocardial infarction. High doses can result in neurological dysfunction, myocardial depression, and depression of the circulatory system. Decreased doses are necessary in liver impairment or in cases of LV dysfunction.

Magnesium

Magnesium sulfate is given in several situations, such as Torsades de pointes (for which it is a first-line agent), low magnesium situations, digoxin toxicity, and to manage post-infarction ventricular arrhythmias. It seems to reduce complications after a myocardial infarction. It also seems to reduce the incidence of supraventricular arrhythmias after an MI.

The dose is given as magnesium sulfate, 1-2 grams IV in 10 milliliters of D5W with a subsequent infusion of 0.5-1 gram per hour. Caution should be given to giving it too rapidly as this can cause hypotension. Calcium can be given as an antidote for an overdose situation. It should be used in lower doses and with caution in those who have severe renal insufficiency.

Procainamide

This is an antiarrhythmic agent use for either ventricular arrhythmias or supraventricular arrhythmias. It suppresses ventricular ectopy, especially when lidocaine has been unsuccessful in controlling the rhythm. It reduces the automaticity of all of the pacemakers in the heart. It is especially useful for recurrent ventricular tachycardia unresponsive to lidocaine.

The loading dose of procainamide is about 15-17 mg/kg IV over thirty minutes (minimum) up to a maximum of 1.5 grams. The infusion should be stopped if there is hypotension or prolongation of the QRS complex by 50 percent of the original length. It can have serious reactions, such as hemolytic anemia, thrombocytopenia, seizures, asystole, or ventricular fibrillation. Typical side effects when given IV include bradycardia, hypertension, urticaria, flushing, and angioedema.

Bretylium

Bretylium is an adrenergic nerve blocking agent that was initially used as an antihypertensive drug. It seems to work synergistically with lidocaine when given for ventricular fibrillation. While lidocaine is the second-line treatment for ventricular fibrillation, bretylium is a good third-line agent. It has positive adrenergic and myocardial effects, causing the release of norepinephrine from adrenergic nerve endings. It lasts about 20 minutes when given in an IV push.

The main indication is ventricular fibrillation, for which it is given at a dose of five milligrams per kilogram IV push and flushed with twenty milliliters of IV fluid. The dose can be increased to 10 milligrams per kilogram IV if the initial dose doesn't work within sixty seconds. Doses can be repeated every six to eight hours. It can take several minutes to take effect, particularly in ventricular tachycardia.

Verapamil and Diltiazem

These are both calcium channel blockers that are rarely associated with ACLS situations, although they do have some usefulness. Both are good antihypertensive agents. Both will cause coronary artery dilatation and decreased oxygen demand on the heart so they can be helpful in a myocardial infarction situation.

The main indication for verapamil is in the treatment of paroxysmal supraventricular tachycardia (PSVT) that doesn't need synchronized cardioversion. It is the second-line treatment after adenosine. It has a direct effect on the AV node, stopping the reentrant pathway. It cannot be used in Wolff-Parkinson-White syndrome as it can lead to ventricular fibrillation.

The dosages of these drugs include giving verapamil at 2.5 to 5 mg IV pushed over one to two minutes, with an effect in three to five minutes. The dosage of diltiazem is 20 mg IV over two minutes or about 0.25 mg/kg IV. When diltiazem is given for atrial flutter, it is given as a bolus over two minutes, followed by an infusion of 5-15 mg/hr, titrated to control the heart rate.

Sodium Bicarbonate

In prolonged cardiac arrest situations, the patient can have metabolic acidosis that adversely affects the cardiac output. Sodium bicarbonate can act as a buffering agent in controlling acidemia in an arrest situation. When it is used for acidosis, the dose is one milliequivalent per kilogram IV bolus every ten minutes. It should be guided by the arterial blood gas determination, if available. The main risk of giving this drug is that it can cause metabolic acidosis. Other risks include hyperosmolality and hypernatremia. It can also inhibit oxygen release in the tissues.

Norepinephrine

This is a naturally-occurring catecholamine similar to epinephrine. It is a positive inotropic and vasopressor drug used in the treatment of shock. It increases systemic vascular resistance, leading to increased blood pressure. It should be used with extreme caution in patients who have ischemic heart disease as it can worsen myocardial ischemia (by increasing the myocardial oxygen demand).

The dose of the drug is 0.5-1.0 micrograms per minute as an IV infusion. It comes in four milliliter ampules that contain 2 mg norepinephrine per ml. It should be mixed in 250 ml of D5W or saline and infused, titrated to the blood pressure. Central intra-arterial blood pressure determinations are preferred over a peripheral blood pressure reading as these determinations are more accurate.

Key Takeaways

- The drug that should be used in almost all ACLS situations is oxygen.
- There are drugs for atrial arrhythmias and ventricular arrhythmias.
- There are several drugs used specifically for improving the blood pressure in shock situations.

Quiz

1. What substance should be given in all ACLS circumstances and is generally given without risk to most patients?
   a. Epinephrine
   b. Oxygen
   c. Norepinephrine
   d. Normal saline

Answer: b. Oxygen is important in nearly all ACLS circumstances and only has to be given with special care to patients with longstanding COPD who will lose their drive to breathe if their O2 sat level is too high.

2. What ACLS drug is primarily used in AV node reentry arrhythmias?
   a. Adenosine
   b. Diltiazem
   c. Epinephrine
   d. Verapamil

Answer: a. Adenosine is especially effective in arrhythmias secondary to AV node reentry pathways. It is especially useful in PSVT, SVT associated with Wolff-Parkinson-White syndrome, and some wide-complex tachycardias.

3. What is the recommended initial dose of adenosine?
   a. 1 mg/kg/minute IV infusion
   b. 12 mg IV push
   c. 6 mg IV push
   d. 6 mg IV or intratracheal

Answer: c. The giving of adenosine requires IV access as the initial dose given is always 6 mg IV given as a fast push into the vein.

4. Dopamine can be given in a range of doses. What is the maximum recommended infusion rate for this drug?
   a. 20 micrograms per kilogram per minute
   b. 10 micrograms per kilogram per minute
   c. 5 micrograms per kilogram per minute
   d. 2 micrograms per kilogram per minute

Answer: a. The maximum recommended dose for an infusion of dopamine is 20 micrograms per kilogram per minute.

5. Which drug is the initial drug of choice for ventricular fibrillation?
   a. Bretylium

b. Epinephrine

c. Atropine

d. Adenosine

Answer: b. The most often used and first-line treatment for ventricular fibrillation is epinephrine.

6. What is the initial dose of epinephrine when given for a cardiac arrest?
    a. 0.1 mg
    b. 0.5 mg
    c. 1 mg
    d. 10 mg

Answer: c. The average dose of epinephrine given in a cardiac arrest situation is 1 mg, which is about 10 ml of a 1: 10,000 solution.

7. What is the recommended dose of magnesium sulfate in an ACLS situation?
    a. 1-2 microgram IV
    b. 1-2 mg IV
    c. 1-2 grams IV
    c. 10-20 grams IV

Answer: c. The dose of magnesium sulfate in an ACLS situation is 1-2 grams IV in 10 ml of D5W.

8. What is the major complication/side effect of a rapid infusion of magnesium sulfate?
    a. Tachyarrhythmia
    b. Hypotension
    c. Frequent PVCs
    d. Oliguria

Answer: b. The major side effect/complication of giving a rapid infusion of magnesium sulfate is hypotension, which is usually transient.

9. The patient is having episodes of recurrent ventricular tachycardia with an inability to suppress the rhythm after giving lidocaine. What is the agent to be given next in most situations?
    a. Bretylium
    b. Atropine
    c. Diltiazem
    d. Procainamide

Answer: d. Procainamide is a good second-line agent in the treatment of recurrent ventricular tachycardia unresponsive to lidocaine.

10. What is the initial dose of choice when giving sodium bicarbonate in an arrest situation?
    a. 1 mEq/kg IV push

b. 1 mEq/kg IV over thirty minutes

c. 10 mEq/kg IV push

d. 10 mEq IV push

Answer: a. The dosage of sodium bicarbonate in an arrest situation is 1 mEq/kg given as an IV push and repeated every ten minutes, guided by the arterial blood gases, if available.

Chapter 8: Pediatric Advanced Life Support

The ACLS guidelines discussed so far have been focused on adults and the common problems seen in adult settings. One of the biggest differences in adult ACLS versus childhood ACLS is that adult ACLS emergencies are usually cardiac in origin, while childhood ACLS emergencies are more respiratory in origin. They experience respiratory failure that leads to deterioration in cardiac function. The drugs and protocols are basically the same but geared toward the child's body.

PALS Basics

Children, fortunately, have a higher survival rate from a cardiorespiratory arrest when compared to adults because they have less irreversible heart disease. In kids, if there is a cardiac arrest, it is almost always secondary to another primary problem. About half of all children with a cardiac arrest will have an initial respiratory arrest that doesn't get adequately treated. The terminal rhythm in children is bradycardia that deteriorates into asystole with the primary cause being hypoxia.

What this means is that prevention is the key feature in treating critically-ill children. Hypoventilation and hypoxic states need to be treated before the cardiac arrest occurs because the outcome is much poorer when the arrest has already happened. The key features in prevention of a cardiac arrest is to maintain oxygenation and adequate ventilations.

Children have a higher oxygen demand and a higher metabolic rate when compared to adults. They develop hypoxemia faster than adults when their airway is compromised or when they stop breathing. They have narrower and shorter airways, meaning that they have an increased risk for airway closure with milder cases of edema of the upper airway.

In intubating children, their vocal cords are positioned such that straight laryngoscopes are preferred over curve-blade laryngoscopes and will provide for the best ability to intubate the child. It may be more difficult to get control over the epiglottis with the laryngoscope blade. The ET tube is often not cuffed in children and infants. Blind placement of the ET tube is not recommended. The airway is shorter so a right mainstem bronchus intubation is more likely.

The child's chest wall is much more compliant than an adult chest wall. What this means is that when positive pressure ventilation is applied (via a bag-valve mask), the chest wall should visibly rise. If this is not the case, it can be assumed that ventilation is not adequate. Lung compliance is low in newborn so more pressure is necessary to ventilate this age group. The respiratory rate for infants and young children is necessarily faster than seen in adults.

The most common tachyarrhythmia seen in children is supraventricular tachycardia with congenital heart disease. Rates are about 180 beats per minute. More commonly, however, is bradycardia secondary to under-ventilation and hypoxia. The finding of bradycardia is ominous and leads to asystole if the hypoxia is not addressed.

Children have the ability to maintain their blood pressure and cardiac output, even with blood loss and other volume loss. They have the capacity to increase their heart rate and will have vasoconstriction to maintain their blood pressure. If they are hypotensive, it can be assumed that their volume loss is extremely serious. When given catecholamines to bring the blood pressure up, children tend to respond greater degrees of tachycardia than is seen in adults.

There may be some difficulty in obtaining IV access in children but, fortunately, if an IV cannot be attained, things like epinephrine can be given via intratracheal instillation or through an intraosseous line, placed in the anterior tibia.

Initial Assessment of the Child in an ALS Situation

As mentioned, one will find ventricular fibrillation as the most common cause of cardiac arrest in adults with a predominance of respiratory failure or trauma as the cause of cardiac arrest in children. When trauma is the cause of the arrest, most patients will be hypovolemic from blood loss and will require volume resuscitation as well as CPR and other ACLS techniques.

When a child is encountered in a cardiac arrest situation or who has the potential to be severely ill, a brief assessment should be undertaken. The child should be evaluated as to having a pulse and respirations. Are the respirations irregular and is the respiratory drive adequate? Is the chest rising and falling with respirations? Obtain a set of vitals, if possible, keeping in mind that the normal child's vital signs are different from adult vital signs.

Vital signs will vary according to age. In infants, the heart rate is about 85-190 (when awake), respiratory rate 30-60 respirations per minute, and temperature of 98.6 degrees Fahrenheit. (There is no need to check a blood pressure in infants). In toddlers and preschoolers, the heart rate is between 98 and 140 bpm, respiratory rate, 22-37 breaths per minute, blood pressure 86-106/42-63, and temperature 98.6 degrees Fahrenheit. School-age children will have vital signs more approaching that of adulthood with a pulse of 75-118 beats per minute, respiratory rate of 18-25 respirations per minute, and a blood pressure of 97-120/57-80.

An overall evaluation of the child's perfusion status takes precedence over the actual vital signs. Check the child's distal pulses and look carefully at their skin color. Cyanosis usually indicates an O2 saturation of less than 94 percent and should be treated immediately with oxygen. Look for the capillary refill of the extremities and at their level of consciousness. These tell a great deal about what the perfusion status is and will be more important assessments than just the vital signs alone.

Look for other signs that the child is critically-ill, such as the presence of seizure activity, petechiae (especially with fever), obvious trauma, or burns greater than ten percent of the body. If any of these signs are present or if there is evidence of poor perfusion, the child probably needs some kind of cardiorespiratory support.

Algorithms for Cardiac Arrest

The pediatric cardiac arrest algorithm is based on the idea that most children will have a respiratory rather than a cardiac cause of their arrest. The successful resuscitation of these children depends most on the delivery of high quality chest compression for the necessary time period for the child to recover. Compressions should not stop at any time unless defibrillation is being performed.

The first step is to recognize that a cardiac arrest is part of the process. CPR should start immediately while the AED is being retrieved. Compressions and ventilations should happen at a 30:2 ratio with a single rescuer or at a 15:2 ratio with two rescuers. The rate should be 100-120 compressions per minute with a depth of greater than a third of the AP chest diameter. CPR should be swapped out for a fresh provider delivering compressions every two minutes. Supplemental oxygen should be part of the ventilatory process and a clear rise in the chest should be visible.

The AED should be applied as soon as it is available and while compressions are ongoing. If there is a shockable rhythm, defibrillation should start at two joules per kilogram with compressions continuing for two minutes after the shock before assessing the patient's pulse. An IV or intraosseous access should next be obtained followed by a shock at four joules per kilogram.

After two shocks and two minutes of CPR after the second shock, IV access should already have been obtained and, if IV access isn't possible, intraosseous access should be obtained by inserting a needle into the anterior tibia. Epinephrine should be given at 0.01 mg/kg every three to five minutes throughout the resuscitation process. After giving a dose of epinephrine, a third shock at 4 joules per kilogram should be performed.

After shocking three times and continuing CPR for two minutes, the child should be reassessed. If they still are in cardiac arrest, the next step is to give either amiodarone 5 mg/kg (given up to three times every few minutes) or lidocaine 1 mg/kg (given once).

If there is no shockable rhythm, CPR should be the mainstay of the resuscitative efforts. An IV or IO access should be obtained with epinephrine given at 0.01 mg/kg every three to five minutes.

There should always be an ongoing search for reversible causes of an arrest situation in children. Reversible causes that can be addressed while CPR and other resuscitation attempts are ongoing include the following:

- Coronary thrombosis
- Pulmonary embolism
- Toxic exposures
- Cardiac tamponade
- Tension pneumothorax
- Hypothermia

- Potassium imbalances (hyperkalemia or hypokalemia)
- Metabolic or respiratory acidosis
- Hypoxia
- Decreased blood volume (blood loss or fluid loss)

Pediatric Bradycardia Algorithm

Because a respiratory arrest and hypoxia are the most common findings in a cardiac arrest situation with children, this bears additional comment and discussion. This is the most likely scenario a provider will encounter in a childhood ACLS situation.

The first thing to do is assess the pulse and determine that the child is bradycardic. The second thing to do is to assess the child's overall level of perfusion. If they are not perfusing and appear in great distress, CPR may be necessary to prevent degeneration into asystole.

Make sure the airway is patent and that the child is breathing adequately. Check the respiratory rate only if the child is otherwise stable. Check an oxygen saturation level and provide oxygen if the O2 saturation is less than 94 percent or the child is dyspneic. A cardiac monitor to evaluate the rhythm should be placed and IV or IO access should be obtained. Only obtain a 12-lead EKG only if the child is stable and treatment is ongoing.

If there is evidence of perfusion, proceed with monitoring. Look for hypotension, altered mental status, or other signs of shock that would indicate the need for further intervention. If there are no signs of perfusion, CPR with oxygen should be given as in an arrest situation. Begin CPR if the pulse is less than 60 bpm and there is evidence of poor perfusion. Atropine should be given at a dose of 0.02 mg/kg up to a maximum single dose of 0.5 mg per dose. If atropine doesn't work, then epinephrine at 0.01 mg/kg, repeated every three to five minutes.

Pediatric Tachycardia Algorithm

The child with tachycardia may or may not be stable. The first step is to assess the patient's vital signs and level of perfusion. Only if the child is not perfusing well or is highly symptomatic should treatment for tachycardia take place.

Oxygen should be started if the child is dyspneic or if the O2 sat is less than 95 percent. The airway should be monitored and kept patent. The vital signs should be monitored as the protocol proceeds. IV or IO access should be obtained and, if the patient is stable, a 12-lead ECG should be obtained.

There are three possible tachycardic rhythms seen in pediatric situations. These include the following:

- **Sinus Tachycardia.** Sinus tachycardia is narrow complex with a typical sinus rhythm pattern on the ECG or rhythm strip. Things like hypovolemia, pain, stress, and dehydration can cause this pattern. The rare is usually less than 220 bpm in infants and less than 180 bpm in older children. The goal for treatment is to find the underlying cause and treat that.

- **Supraventricular tachycardia.** In this situation, the P waves are either absent or do not look normal. The rate is greater than 220 bpm in infants and greater than 180 bpm in older children. The treatment is to give adenosine at 0.1 mg/kg as a rapid bolus, repeating the dose a second time at 0.2 mg/kg IV push. If this does not work, try synchronized cardioversion (under sedation if possible) at 0.5-1.0 Joules per kilogram first, followed by synchronized cardioversion at 2 joules/kg.
- **Wide complex tachycardia.** In such cases the QRS complex is greater than 0.9 seconds and often looks abnormal. This is probably ventricular tachycardia and should be treated as such. Any hypotensive child or a child with an altered level of consciousness should be shocked immediately with synchronized cardioversion at 0.5 joules per kilogram (first try) and 2 joules per kilogram (second and subsequent tries). If the child isn't hypotensive, adenosine should be tried at 0.1 mg/kg (up to 6 mg) first dose, followed by adenosine 0.2 mg/kg (up to 12 mg) second dose—both given by IV rapid push. If the child still has this rhythm but is not hypotensive, the third-line treatments include amiodarone 5 mg/kg IV over 20-60 minutes or procainamide 15 mg IV over 30-60 minutes. These two drugs cannot be given together.

Algorithm for Pediatric Respiratory Emergencies

Respiratory emergencies are perhaps the most common ACLS situation (along with bradycardia) in children. Once beginning care for a child with a potential respiratory emergency, it is important to start with the basic protocol, which includes positioning for the easiest breathing, suctioning, pulse oximetry evaluation (and giving oxygen for dyspnea or an O2 sat less than 94 percent), ECG monitoring, and basic life support measures.

The additional treatment depends on what is causing the respiratory emergency. Some basic treatments include the following:

- **Anaphylaxis.** Give IM or SQ epinephrine, albuterol, antihistamines, and steroids.
- **Croup.** Give nebulized racemic epinephrine and IV steroids.
- **Foreign body aspiration.** Give basic airway support and contact an expert who can remove the foreign body via a bronchoscope.
- **Asthma attack.** Give albuterol with or without ipatropium as an initial treatment, followed by steroids, subcutaneous epinephrine, terbutaline (by any route), and magnesium sulfate.
- **Bronchiolitis.** Give bronchodilating medications and perform regular nasal suctioning.
- **Pulmonary edema.** Intubate if needed and provide oxygen with PEEP (positive end-expiratory pressure), diuretic therapy to draw fluid off the lungs, and vasoactive drugs if the child is hypotensive.
- **Pneumonia.** Support with oxygen, antibiotics, nebulized albuterol, and possibly CPAP (continuous positive airway pressure).

- **Poisoning with disordered breathing.** Call poison control for antidotes if available. Support breathing with a patent airway and intubation/oxygen if necessary.
- **Neuromuscular disease.** These children often need ventilation support with intubation and a ventilator until their condition resolves.
- **Head injury.** These children have breathing disorders because of increased intracranial pressure. They need to be hyperventilated, well-oxygenated, and should be kept cool as high temperatures can worsen their outcome.

Key Takeaways

- Pediatric Advanced Life Support involves the resuscitation and management of pediatric cardiorespiratory emergencies.
- Most children's cardiac arrests start with hypoxia that leads to bradycardia, which degenerates into asystole.
- Children have more respiratory arrests than cardiac arrests.
- Children may have tachycardia or bradycardia from various reasons.

Quiz

1. What is the main difference between pediatric ACLS emergencies and adult ACLS emergencies?
   a. Children often require more drug therapies.
   b. Children suffer from respiratory emergencies more than cardiac emergencies.
   c. Most childhood ACLS emergencies are from congenital heart diseases.
   d. Children have more hypotensive emergencies than adults.

Answer: b. Children suffer from more respiratory ACLS emergencies than adults, who suffer from more cardiac emergencies.

2. What is the most common terminal rhythm seen in cardiac arrest cases in children?
   a. Severe bradycardia leading to asystole
   b. Paroxysmal supraventricular tachycardia
   c. Ventricular fibrillation
   d. Third-degree heart block

Answer: a. The most common terminal rhythm seen in children suffering from a cardiac arrest is severe bradycardia that degenerates into asystole.

3. What is not a major difference in the intubation of a child over an adult?
   a. They have a shorter airway so right mainstem bronchial intubation is more likely.
   b. It is more difficult to have control over the epiglottis.
   c. The ET tube is narrower.
   d. A curved laryngoscope blade is preferred over a straight laryngoscope blade.

Answer: d. The truth is that a straight laryngoscope blade is preferred over a curved laryngoscope blade because of the placement of the child's vocal cords.

4. What is true of assessing the vital signs and assessing perfusion in children?
   a. The blood pressure needs to be assessed in infants using a leg cuff.
   b. The vital signs give an accurate impression of the child's level of perfusion.
   c. Abnormal signs of perfusion should take precedence over the actual vital signs.
   d. There is no need to check the vital signs if a thorough assessment of perfusion is performed.

Answer: c. If a child shows abnormal signs of perfusion, this takes precedence over the actual vital signs obtained.

5. What thing best represents the cornerstone of the successful pediatric ACLS resuscitation?
   a. Delivering high quality chest compressions until the child is resuscitated.
   b. Using antiarrhythmics and vasopressors intravenously or through an intraosseous line.
   c. Delivering an adequate number of ventilations per minute.
   d. Monitoring and maintaining the blood pressure through volume resuscitation.

Answer: a. The cornerstone of successful ACLS resuscitation in children is the delivery of quality chest compressions until the child is resuscitated.

6. During a pediatric resuscitation, when can compressions stop?
   a. When the IV is being started and during defibrillation
   b. When respirations/ventilations are being delivered
   c. At no time should the compressions be stopped
   d. Compressions should only be stopped during defibrillation

Answer: d. Compressions should be stopped only during defibrillation but should go on at all other times until the child recovers or until the efforts have been spent and the child has no chance of recovery.

7. The child with bradycardia is the most common ACLS situation the provider will find in pediatric advance life support. What pulse is the lowest acceptable rate in children?
   a. 80 bpm
   b. 60 bpm
   c. 40 bpm
   d. 30 bpm

Answer: b. A pulse rate of less than 60 bpm is considered a bradycardic rhythm in children and adults alike.

8. In the pediatric bradycardia algorithm, if the child is bradycardic and there is no perfusion, what drug should be given first?
    a. Epinephrine
    b. Procainamide
    c. Bretylium
    d. Atropine

Answer: d. Once an IV access has been obtained, it is a good idea to give atropine if the child has bradycardia but isn't perfusing after oxygenation. The dose is 0.02 mg/kg up to 0.5 mg per dose.

9. Which is not considered a typical tachycardic rhythm seen in children?
    a. Sinus tachycardia
    b. Torsades de pointes
    c. Supraventricular tachycardia
    d. Wide-complex tachycardia

Answer: b. All of the above are common causes of pediatric tachycardia except for Torsades de pointes, which would be extremely uncommon.

10. What is the first treatment recommended for a child with an asthma attack and respiratory distress?
    a. Terbutaline
    b. Subcutaneous epinephrine
    c. Nebulized albuterol
    d. IV steroids

Answer: c. The initial treatment of choice is nebulized albuterol with or without also using ipratropium. The other choices are second and third-line treatments.

Chapter 9: Prehospital Trauma Assessment

The care of the trauma patient in Advanced Trauma Life Support (ATLS) begins with the prehospital care. Trauma patients can be anywhere from remote rural locations and farm injuries to urban gang locations and gunshots. Either way, it is up to the prehospital team to evaluate and quickly manage these patients until they reach definitive care at the hospital. Prehospital assessment and management of the trauma patient is the focus of this chapter.

Initial Assessment of the Trauma Patient

The initial management of the trauma patient requires the quick assessment of major injuries and the institution of whatever life-saving treatment that can be given under the circumstances. Timing is critical in the care of a traumatically-injured patient so the initial assessment must start with the following:

- Preparing the scene so that it is safe for victims and rescuers alike.
- Triage so that the people likely to survive with the most severe injuries are treated first. This may mean passing up a patient who is extremely injured because their chance of survival is zero.
- Primary survey of airway, breathing, circulation, disability, and exposure.
- Resuscitation of injured patients.
- Adjuncts to the resuscitation and primary survey.
- Deciding on patient's mode of transfer and speed of transfer.
- Secondary survey completion.
- Adjuncts to the secondary survey.
- Continued monitoring and reevaluation after resuscitation.
- Transfer to definitive care.

It should be noted that the primary and secondary surveys are not just single events but should be repeated often enough to be able to identify any specific changes that require ongoing or additional intervention.

In clinical practice, the resuscitation, primary survey, and even the secondary surveys are done simultaneously or at least, in parallel to one another. During this time, the provider uses their best judgment to determine which procedures need to be done in the field and which can wait until the patient arrives at the hospital.

Coordination between the prehospital team and the hospital emergency department is crucial so that the incoming hospital can be prepared to quickly further manage the patient's care once they arrive at the emergency room. Usually, this is accomplished via an ambulance-to-hospital communication system but can be done with just cell phones.

The main emphasis on the prehospital care is airway maintenance, control of external bleeding, and management of shock. If these three things are handled correctly, the patient will survive their prehospital phase and will arrive in reasonable shape when the hospital/emergency department team takes over. The patient should be immobilized for protection of their spine and prepared for transport.

Every effort should be made to keep the scene time as short as possible as the patient's true definitive treatment will happen at the emergency department. The time spent at the scene should be devoted to taking care of those things that would be lethal prior to the patient's arrival at the hospital.

The initial assessment should also include an attempt to understand the mechanism of injury as this is something that can only be understood by seeing the vehicles that were in a crash or the height of the patient's fall. This needs to be relayed to the hospital staff as a part of the report given when the patient gets to the emergency department.

Steps to the Approach of the Trauma Patient

Before even assessing the patient, the first thing the provider needs to do is size up the scene. In a car accident scene, there will likely be cars and trucks traveling by on the road where the provider is attempting to treat patients so care must be taken to make sure no one at the scene—providers, bystanders, and patients—are in danger during the treatment time. If there are hazardous materials or live electrical wires, this needs to be addressed before caring for the patient.

Get a general assessment of the scene. How serious is the automobile damage? How high was the patient's fall? What type of crush injury did the patient sustain? Was there deployment of the airbag or was the patient ejected? All of these impressions will help the care of the patient and should be conveyed to the hospital crew.

- The first thing to do as part of sizing up the scene is to practice body substance isolation precautions. It means wearing gloves when blood is present and using an Ambu bag (bag-valve-mask) in order to ventilate the patient without having to do mouth-to-mouth resuscitation.

- The second thing to do is make the scene safe for everyone. Put up cones so cars don't travel where you are treating the patient. Make sure electricity in live and exposed wires is turned off. Make sure there are no hazardous materials present that might affect the rescuers or the victims.

- Determine the mechanism of injury. Take a look at the scene from the perspective of a sleuth trying to determine what happened and how severe to expect the victims' injuries to be. The vehicle will be important to look at in an automobile accident to see how damaged it was. Get an estimate of the speeds involved in the crash as this will clue the rescuers and hospital staff in as to what injuries to expect in the victims.

- Determine the number of patients you are dealing with and triage them in as short a time as possible. Victims that are not expected to survive regardless of aggressive treatment may be passed up in lieu of treating the patients that will respond best to treatment but that will need the fastest intervention. Victims that are stable at the scene can simply be transported without a lot of intervention as they will survive the trip to definitive care at the hospital.

- Immobilize the cervical spine. Unless the mechanism of injury is obviously not at all likely to injure the cervical spine, the immobilization of the cervical spine is crucial and should be done first. Resuscitation itself can cause movement of the cervical spine so consideration to immobilizing it first should be undertaken before any other treatment.

Sizing up the scene takes just a minute or so but is important to do before getting into the initial assessment of the victims. The scene should be assessed and controlled as soon as the rescuers arrive on the scene. Hopefully, there will be enough personnel to treat the patients as well as keep the scene secure.

First Impressions

After the scene is secure, it is time to get a first impression of the victim. Are they sick, not sick, or unclear as to their status? While doing this, the cervical spine should be immobilized so that resuscitative attempts don't cause quadriplegia or other neurological injury to the victim. Determine the victim's level of consciousness and get a quick Glasgow coma scale evaluation out of the victim.

Airway, breathing, and circulation are the next steps of the impression. An awake patient and an unconscious patient both can have problems with these three things so, after determining the level of consciousness of the patient, the ABCs are crucial to do. This involves doing a jaw-thrust maneuver on patients who don't appear to be breathing and then assessing the quality and quantity of the breaths. Is the chest rising and falling? What is their approximate breathing rate? Breathing too fast (more than 35 breaths per minute) or too slow (less than 8 breaths per minute) may indicate that the patient needs to be ventilated. This usually involves a bag-valve mask and high flow oxygen.

The third step Is the pulse. The radial artery in the wrist is appropriate for all adults who are conscious, while an unresponsive adult should have the pulse checked at the carotid artery. Infants and small children should have their pulse checked at the brachial artery at the elbow. After checking the pulse, look for obvious signs of bleeding and make attempts to control it. If there is no pulse or if the heart rate is less than sixty in children, CPR is recommended.

Generally, more than one rescuer is necessary to treat one critically-ill victim as this provides the fastest and most effective way to manage these types of patients. One rescuer can get a history and assess the scene, while another is getting vital signs and doing the primary survey. With enough rescuers, the scene assessment, patient initial assessment, the primary survey, and immobilizing the patient should all take less than ten minutes.

Getting a SAMPLE History

If the patient or patient representative is available, a SAMPLE history should be obtained. This is a focused history that will give the rescuer the basic information necessary to quickly manage the patient. The information gotten through the SAMPLE history should be part of the documentation done upon transfer of the patient to the hospital.

The SAMPLE history evaluates these things:

- S—Signs and symptoms the patient has
- A—Allergies to medications, latex, or other substances
- M—Medications the patient is taking
- P—Past illnesses, such as diabetes, heart disease, cancer, or other major illnesses
- L—Last oral intake
- E—Events leading up to the injury

Obtaining a Revised Trauma Score

The revised trauma score is a way to objectively assess each victim in a traumatic situation. It is a simple measurement that can be passed on to the hospital staff as a way of determining exactly how sick the trauma patient is.

There are three aspects to the revised trauma score: the Glasgow Coma Scale determination, the systolic blood pressure, and the victim's respiratory rate. The score range is 0-12, with higher numbers indicating a patient who is in better shape than a patient with a lower score. Patients with a score of 12 can have delayed treatment. Patients with a score of 11 need urgent treatment. Patients with a score of 3-10 need immediate treatment. People with a score of less than 3 are generally dead or terminal and should not receive priority care as they are not likely to survive. Figure 15 describes the revised trauma score:

Revised Trauma Score					
Glasgow Coma scale		Systolic Blood Pressure		Respiratory Rate	
GCS	RTS score	SBP	RTS score	RR	RTS score
13-15	4	>89	4	10-29	4
9-12	3	76-89	3	>29	3
6-8	2	50-75	2	6-9	2
4-5	1	1-49	1	1-5	1
3	0	0	0	0	0

Ongoing assessment should happen after assessing the patient the first time and after the patient has been packaged for transport. These patients may have internal injuries or head injuries that cannot immediately be seen but that will affect the patient over a period of time. Patient with a head injury can lose consciousness or can stop breathing because of herniation of the brain through the foramen magnum. For this reason, continual assessment of the patient should happen throughout the care and transfer of the patient.

Documentation and Communication

Most EMS systems have dedicated channels to communicate between ambulances and to the hospital. EMS care providers/rescuers should always keep everyone informed as to where they are and what they are doing. The status of the patient, and any changes in the patient's vitals and clinical situation should be transmitted via a dedicated MED channel. In some cases, the communication can be a two-way situation in which the emergency medical doctor can provide helpful information and orders to the rescuer that can help the patient in the field.

With each interaction with a victim, even those that aren't transported by ambulance, a Patient Care Report or PCR should be done. The patient's name, age, address, time of treatment, complaint, physical exam results, and any treatments given are a part of this record. These are legal medical records that could come up later in a legal situation, especially in things like car accidents that later have legal action taken against the responsible party.

It is important to document everything that is observed and done. The inadequate PCR may later be scrutinized negatively in court or by lawyers, especially if the patient has a serious injury or does not survive the accident. The document should be objective and should not contain assumptions about the patient or the situation involved. Things like "whose fault the accident was" should not be part of the PCR as this is not an expectation of a trauma care provider.

Transferring the Patient

Part of the care of the trauma patient is making the assessment of where to take the critically-injured patient. There are different levels of trauma centers. Sometimes, the closest hospital is not the hospital to send the patient to because it is not at a level appropriate for the patient's injuries. Severely injured patients often do better at trauma centers better able to manage their unique needs than they do at just any hospital.

The following is a summary of what each level means:

- Level I Trauma Center—this has the highest level of service and the most resources, including emergency surgery services, in order to treat the critically-ill patient. They have a high level of staff education, trauma leadership, and research related to trauma care. They have 24-hour in-house surgical care and fast availability of specialist care.
- Level II Trauma Center—these offer basically the same level of care as the Level I trauma center but are generally not involved in education or research and simply have staff doctors and resources available to treat the patient. They may not have all of the surgical specialties or other specialists quickly available but offer 24-hours emergency services.

- Level III Trauma Center—these can assess patients, resuscitate patients, and have surgical services close at hand but not necessarily in-house. They have agreements for transfer of more critically-ill patients to a Level I or Level II Trauma Center. They have outreach programs and preventative programs in the community.
- Level IV Trauma Center—these have an ability to provide ATLS services before transferring those that are critically-ill to a higher-level trauma center. They don't usually have trauma surgeons readily available but can care for injured patients according to ATLS protocols. They offer 24-hour emergency services.
- Level V Trauma Center—this may or may not provide 24-hour services. They have the ability to evaluate, stabilize, and diagnose ailments in most patients who have been injured but the major goal is to send these patients for definitive care/surgical intervention at a higher-level trauma center.

The Secondary Survey

After the primary survey and initial resuscitative efforts have been done, the secondary survey should be undertaken if the patient is stable enough and if time allows. The secondary survey becomes a head-to-toe evaluation of the patient's overall status. The following things are part of the secondary survey:

- Scalp evaluation for bruising, depressions, or lacerations
- Mouth evaluation for lacerations
- Teeth for loss of teeth
- Nose for deformities or bleeding
- Ears for CSF or blood loss
- Eyes for penetrating injuries or foreign bodies
- Jaw for malocclusion
- Cervical spine for tenderness or deformity
- Trachea for deviation or crepitus
- Chest wall for bruising
- Lung fields for aeration
- Heart sounds for murmurs or other abnormal sounds
- Abdominal examination for penetrating injuries, tenderness, bowel sounds, or pelvic pain
- Limbs for joint injuries or bony injuries and lacerations
- Back for lacerations, bruising, or bony tenderness
- Buttocks for bruising or lacerations
- Perineum for lacerations or bruising
- Genitalia for bleeding or trauma

Key Takeaways

- The first thing to assess in a trauma situation is the scene.
- The first thing to assess with regard to the patient is their level of consciousness.
- The Revised Trauma Score includes an assessment of the Glasgow Coma Score, respiratory rate, and systolic blood pressure.
- The patient needs to be transferred to the highest-level trauma center appropriate or the patient's injuries.

Quiz

1. What is the first step in dealing with a trauma situation?
   a. Triaging the patients.
   b. Assessing the sickest patient first.
   c. Making sure the scene is safe for everyone.
   d. Reducing exposure to the victim.

Answer: c. The first thing that must be done is securing the scene to make sure the situation is safe for both the victims and the rescuers.

2. What is not a part of the prehospital team's major focuses?
   a. Pain control
   b. Airway management
   c. Control of external bleeding
   d. Shock management

Answer: a. The three main goals of prehospital care include airway management, control of external bleeding, and shock management. Pain control is not part of prehospital goals.

3. You are caring for a patient ejected from a motor vehicle. Upon reaching the patient, what is the first intervention you should consider?
   a. Starting a large-bore IV.
   b. Getting a quick set of vitals.
   c. Tilting back the head and opening the airway.
   d. Immobilizing the cervical spine.

Answer: d. A victim likely to have a cervical spine injury should have their cervical spine immobilized before attempting to work on the patient. It takes just seconds to do and may save the patient's neurological status.

4. At what heart rate in a child or below should CPR commence in a trauma situation?
   a. Seventy bpm
   b. Sixty bpm

c. Fifty bpm

d. Forty bpm

Answer: b. At a heart rate of below 60 bpm in a child, the rescuer should commence doing CPR as this rate is ineffective in perfusing the victim.

5. What assessment is not a part of the SAMPLE history?
   a. Allergies
   b. Address
   c. Medications
   d. Signs and symptoms

Answer: b. The SAMPLE history includes all of the above things except for the patient's address, which can be gotten at a later time when billing becomes important. It should not be part of the patient's initial evaluation.

6. Which Revised Trauma Score on a victim would indicate the need for immediate treatment?
   a. Twelve
   b. Eleven
   c. Seven
   d. Two

Answer: c. The patient with a Revised Trauma Score of 3-10 need immediate treatment. Patients with a score of eleven need urgent treatment; patients with a score of twelve can have delayed treatment; patients with a score of less than three are not likely to survive and should be passed up.

7. What is not included in the assessment of a patient receiving a Revised Trauma Score?
   a. Glasgow Coma Scale
   b. Respiratory rate
   c. Systolic blood pressure
   d. Pulse rate

Answer: d. The pulse rate is not a part of the Revised Trauma Score; however, the other three things are included.

8. What item should not be part of the Patient Care Record?
   a. The patient's vital signs
   b. An assessment of who was at fault in the accident
   c. The treatments given to the patient
   d. The patient's name and address

Answer: b. This is a legal document that should be completely objective. It is not the job of the healthcare provider to make assumptions about who was at fault in the accident or any other assumptions that cannot be objectively proven.

9. At which hospital/trauma center would an in-house trauma surgeon be available to treat injured patients?
   a. Level I
   b. Level II
   c. Level IV
   d. Level V

Answer: a. A Level I trauma center is most likely has an in-house trauma surgeon available on a 24-hour-a-day basis to treat critically-injured patients.

10. What is not part of the secondary survey?
    a. Scalp evaluation
    b. Bone evaluation of limbs
    c. Back evaluation for lacerations
    d. Airway evaluation for patency

Answer: d. The airway evaluation is part of the primary survey and not the secondary survey. The other items are a part of the secondary survey.

Chapter 10: ATLS Protocols for Adults

One of the newest programs to come out of the need for better and more consistent protocols for the critically-ill patient is ATLS or Advanced Trauma Life Support. This is a provider training program that is specifically directed at caring for the trauma patient. The protocols were first developed and are revised periodically by the American College of Surgeons. It is directed at all types of healthcare providers—from prehospital rescuers to emergency medical doctors. The focus of this chapter is on ATLS for adults and the protocols involved.

Airway and Ventilation Management

The fastest way to kill the injured patient is to inadequately oxygenate them. Oxygenation begins with a patent airway so, upon seeing the injured patient and determining their level of consciousness, the airway must be evaluated and managed. In the situation of an injured patient with a possible cervical spine injury, the head must be kept in alignment and the jaw-thrust maneuver must be done in order to open the airway.

The decision must be made as to how to ventilate the patient. An unconscious patient should be intubated or provided with a cricothyrotomy (if there is facial trauma precluding oral intubation). If intubation fails or is not felt to be necessary, high flow oxygen must be provided with an Ambu bag or another bag-valve mask device. Intubation is preferred in the unconscious or semi-conscious patient because these people may have just eaten and will have a high risk of aspirating the stomach contents in vomiting—even while they are unconscious. If giving O2 by mask in a conscious patient, it should be high flow oxygen at 100 percent.

Consideration should be made to inserting an orogastric or nasogastric tube in order to aspirate stomach contents and air in the stomach. Providing this will make respirations more successful because the stomach isn't filled and pushing up on the lungs and aspiration of stomach contents will be less likely. Most patients aren't intubated immediately so they can have excess air in the stomach from initial bag-valve mask breathing.

Recognize that the patient may have neck, maxillofacial, or laryngeal trauma that will both obstruct the airway and make it more difficult to establish an airway by mean of an endotracheal (ET) tube. This is where it pays to learn how to perform cricothyrotomy in order to ventilate patient with severe facial or laryngeal trauma.

The best way to evaluate the patient's airway patency is to simple talk to the patient. The patient who I talking usually has a patent airway and might be ventilating adequately, although this should be assessed by evaluating the patient's overall clinical status, including looking for cyanosis or getting an oxygen saturation level.

Besides the unconscious patient, those who are obtunded because of intoxication by alcohol or drugs, patients with head and neck trauma that might swell over time and obstruct the airway, and patients with thoracic trauma need to be intubated for the best oxygenation. An oxygen-enriched source of O2 should be given, preferably 100 percent oxygen.

Head injury patients have a specific reason why they should be intubated. Head injuries can cause a mass effect in the brain from bleeding or swelling of the brain. Increased intracranial pressure can cause herniation of the brain through the foramen magnum, which can shut off the respiratory drive to breathe. Hypercarbia makes this problem more likely so, intubating and hyperventilating these patients can decrease their intracranial pressure.

All patients who have suffered trauma are at a high risk for vomiting and, if they are obtunded or unconscious (or just lying on their back), they are at a high aspiration risk. As mentioned, an orogastric or nasogastric tube can help if this is available. A simple thing that can be done if a nasogastric tube is not available is to roll the patient on their side to decrease the risk of aspirating their stomach contents. Suctioning, if available, should be handy to clear out the nose and mouth if necessary.

The most important thing to do in obtaining an airway in the severely-injured patient with neck and/or facial trauma is to do it quickly with direct visualization of the vocal cords. The anatomy may be displaced so the vocal cords might be in a different position than is expected. For this reason, when placing the ET tube, the vocal cords should be visualized.

Evidence of upper airway obstruction include an unwillingness to lie down, subcutaneous air in the neck, the finding of a palpable anterior neck fracture, and hoarseness of the voice. Swelling can be rapid and can obstruct the airway quickly so these patients need a definitive airway as soon as possible. Doing flexible endoscopic intubation may be helpful in visualizing the vocal cords directly. If this is not possible, a cricothyrotomy should be considered.

In evaluating the ventilatory status of the patient, the first thing to do is to assess the patient's level of activity and degree of consciousness. A patient who is agitated may have hypoxia needing oxygen and possible ventilatory support. An obtunded patient may have hypercarbia, necessitating ventilatory support. Cyanosis suggests hypoxemia. Hypoxemia can also be assessed by looking at the nail beds and the skin around the mouth. These are late findings of hypoxia so this is why doing an ongoing oxygen saturation level is preferred.

If the airway is open, the next step is to determine if the patient is ventilating. CNS depression, chest wall trauma, decreased or increased respiratory rate, or shallow breathing are all things that can lead to under-ventilation even with a patent airway. Even belligerence and angry outburst might indicate a hypoxic patient who is not ventilating properly. People with preexisting lung disease are at risk for ventilatory failure (even with minor trauma) and an injury to the cervical spine can adversely affect the patient's ability to take an adequate breath because they will have paralyzed breathing muscles.

Besides the oxygen saturation level, which is crucial in identifying hypoxemia in the trauma patient, an end-tidal CO_2 level should be done to see if the patient is ventilating adequately. The exam can help. Look for symmetry of breathing and the presence of good breath sounds on both sides of the chest. Rapid breathing can indicate respiratory distress just as much as slow breathing.

Special care must be taken when intubating the patient with possible cervical spine injury. The neck must be immobilized by a second person and intubation must take place with the neck and head in alignment. The typical "tilting-back" of the head cannot happen when a C-spine injury is suspected. The jaw, however, can be thrust forward and intubation can still take place (but with some difficulty).

An oropharyngeal airway can help keep the airway open with an Ambu bag ventilating the patient. It is ideal to use a tongue depressor to prevent the tongue from falling back and obstructing the airway, making it difficult to put the airway in. It can't be used in conscious patients as they will gag and/or vomit—increasing the aspiration risk.

A nasopharyngeal airway can be used in conscious or semiconscious patients. It cannot be used when a cribriform plate fracture is suspected as the tube could pass through the plate and get into the brain tissue. It should be lubricated well and put gently in the nostril that appears the easiest to pass the tube through.

The laryngeal mask airway or LMA can be used on a temporary basis in those patients who cannot be intubated. It is not a definitive airway and must be replaced by an ET tube in the emergency department. There is an ILMA, which is an intubating LMA that allows for intubating the patient through the LMA device after reaching the emergency department.

The laryngeal tube airway or LTA is done without visualization of the glottis and doesn't require placing the head or neck in any particular position. It is also not a definitive airway and plans for a definitive airway (probably an ET tube) should be made as soon as the LTA is inserted. It can buy time to get the patient oxygenated until the patient reaches the ED. The major advantage of this airway is that it doesn't require as much skill as placing an ET tube.

There two ports in the LTA device. The first enters the esophagus and the second enters the airway but it isn't immediately clear as to which one is which. The rescuer must determine which port inflates the lungs and must use that port only while occluding the non-functional port with a balloon. A CO_2 detector can be used to make the determination as to which port to occlude and which port to ventilate.

The definition of a definitive airway is a device that has a tube in the trachea with the cuff inflated below the vocal cord and having this device attached to a high-flow oxygen source. If a multilumen esophageal airway is placed, it must be removed completely to get a definitive airway in place. The endotracheal tube is the safest and best way to have a definitive airway for the trauma patient.

There are three main reasons why a definitive airway should be established in a trauma patient:

- Inability to have a good, patent airway by any other means with a potential for compromise of the airway because of the patient's medical condition.
- Breathing difficulties, such as apnea, under-ventilation.
- Disability problems, which basically means the patient has a head injury that causes them to under-ventilate and possibly develop hypercarbia. A Glasgow Coma Scale score of eight or less indicates the need for ventilation with an ET tube and high flow oxygen.

When ventilating the patient, sedation and muscle relaxants, along with pain medication, may be necessary to continue an ET tube ventilation, especially in the critically-injured patient who is not completely unconscious but needs definitive ventilatory support. If the need for urgent intubation isn't there, a set of cervical spine x-rays or CT scan of the cervical spine should be done before placing the ET tube.

Nasotracheal tube is a second choice over the oropharyngeal ET tube. There can be sinusitis or pressure necrosis of the nasal passages if the nasotracheal tube is left in too long and it can't be done if there is a possible fracture of the facial bones, frontal sinus fracture, cribriform plate fracture, or basilar skull fracture. Patients with CSF leaks of the ears or nose, or patients with raccoon's eyes or a positive Battle's sign, should be considered to have a basilar skull fracture and shouldn't have a nasopharyngeal tube placed.

Rapid sequence intubation (RSI) is recommended for all trauma patients because they do not always have empty stomachs and may aspirate. A plan should be in place as to what to do if the technique fails. A high flow oxygen source should be ready and suction should be available. The patient should be preoxygenated with 100 percent O2 before intubation. About 1-2 mg of succinylcholine should be given along with etomidate, which is a good induction drug. The succinylcholine relaxes the muscles, effectively paralyzing the patient. Other sedating methods, such as propofol or Fentanyl can be used prior to giving the paralytic agent. Once these are given, cricoid pressure is applied and the tube is passed. If possible, a CO2 detector should be applied to affirm that the tube is in the trachea.

The Management of Shock

The main cause of shock in the trauma patient is blood loss but later shock can develop secondary to infection. There is no good test that can prove shock. It is based on the clinical findings indicating a reduced perfusion of the body. The definition of shock is determined by the finding of poor perfusion and oxygenation of the end-organs, including the liver, kidneys, intestines, brain, and distal extremities.

After shock is identified, the cause of the shock should be determined. Hypovolemia from blood loss is the main cause of shock in the trauma patient but other options include cardiogenic shock, neurogenic shock, septic shock, or obstructive shock. A tension pneumothorax can cause obstructive shock as can cardiac tamponade. Neurogenic shock results from severe damage to the cervical or thoracic spine, causing neurogenic vasodilation. Septic shock is rare but can be seen in patients who present to the emergency department after a several-hour delay in transport since the trauma.

It is important to remember that, at any given point in time, about seventy percent of the total blood volume will be in the veins so a loss of volume affects the venous pressure and the venous return in the heart. This pressure drives amount of blood filling the ventricles and the ultimate cardiac output. The cardiac pump needs blood in order to have a cardiac output and, without that, the patient's blood pressure drops and there is lack of end-organ tissue perfusion.

The early responses to blood loss include constriction of the blood vessels going to the skin, viscera, and muscle so that blood flow can be maintained as much as possible to the heart, brain, and kidneys. The heart rate will increase in order to preserve a normal cardiac output.

This means that tachycardia may be the first sign that blood loss is occurring and shock is possible. There is a release of endogenous catecholamines that increase the peripheral vascular resistance—increasing diastolic blood pressure but not much affecting the end-organ perfusion. Histamine, cytokines, bradykinin, and beta-endorphins are released, affecting the vascular permeability and microcirculation of the tissues.

The best way to restore adequate cardiac output and perfusion of the end organs is to improve venous return by stopping the bleeding source and providing IV fluids. This prevents the conversion of circulation from aerobic metabolism to anaerobic metabolism. If shock is allowed to go on for very long, ATP (adenosine triphosphate) levels decrease and the normal electrical gradient of the cells is disrupted. Proinflammatory mediators are released, resulting in the end-organ dysfunction and end-organ death that is seen in shock.

The loss of blood volume fluid through tissue swelling and a lack of cellular permeability makes the blood loss and hypoperfusion worse, increasing the amount of fluid necessary for the resuscitation of the trauma patient in shock. Vasopressors cannot be given in blood-loss shock because it only worsens the perfusion of the end-organs. The treatment of choice is isotonic saline or other isotonic fluid, with blood provision the ultimate end-goal, even though that is often delayed until the patient has been resuscitated with IV fluids.

A good fluid resuscitation involves giving a warmed isotonic electrolyte solution, such as normal saline or lactated Ringer's solution. These will expand the intravascular volume. About one to two liters should quickly be given if shock is recommended in adults and 20 ml/kg IV fluid bolus should be given to children with shock. After this, the clinical state of the patient monitors the IV rate given. Urinary output is a good measurement of the resuscitative efforts and should be regularly monitored with a Foley catheter in place. Remember that, unless the patient has surgery or obvious resolution of bleeding from an external source, they will continue to bleed and will continue to need fluids.

Persistently giving fluids, however, is not a good substitute for surgery to find and stop the bleeding. Just giving crystalloid to bring the blood pressure up will increase the bleeding rate and will cause hypothermia, acidosis, and blood clotting problems. This is why giving blood, fresh frozen plasma, and platelets may be necessary in patients who have lost a lot of blood and still hover in the area of "shock" despite giving large amounts of isotonic fluids. One thing that can help offset this problem is to aim for a slightly hypotensive state that helps perfusion but doesn't cause such an increase in blood pressure that bleeding is made worse.

Urinary output, as mentioned, is a good measurement of blood flow to the kidneys. When the Foley catheter is placed, the goal should include a urinary output of 0.5 ml/kg/hr in adults and 1 mg/kg/hr in children above the age of one. About 2 mg/kg/hr is an appropriate urinary output for children under the age of one year being evaluated for their response to getting IV fluids or blood. Ideally, any blood given should be type-specific but, if the patient is bleeding out and time is a factor, O-negative blood can be given.

Patients who do not respond to fluid resuscitation should be further evaluated for the possibility of having non-hemorrhagic shock, such as a cardiac tamponade or tension pneumothorax. Placing a central line and following the jugular venous pressure (JVP) may easily tell the difference between hemorrhagic shock and non-hemorrhagic shock.

Key Takeaways

- The patient with trauma first needs to have their airway managed and maintained patent throughout the resuscitative process.
- A patient can have a patent airway but may still require ventilatory support because they aren't ventilating for a variety of reasons.
- The first sign of shock in the patient with hemorrhagic shock is tachycardia.
- A warmed bolus of isotonic crystalloid solution is the first treatment modality in the management of shock.

Quiz

1. What is the preferred way of giving oxygen in the unconscious trauma patient?
   a. High flow oxygen via an endotracheal tube
   b. High flow oxygen via a nasal cannula at 4 liters per minute
   c. Bag-valve mask
   d. 100 percent O2 by facial mask

Answer: a. An endotracheal tube should be considered in the unconscious patient because it protects the airway from aspiration and provides a high flow oxygen.

2. If using a mask on a breathing trauma patient, what amount of oxygen do you want to provide them with?
   a. 1 liter per minute
   b. 2 liters per minute
   c. 4 liters per minute
   d. High flow of 100 percent O2

Answer: d. When using a mask in a trauma patient, the oxygen should be set at 100 percent and delivered using a high flow.

3. What is the main advantage of using an ET tube to ventilate the trauma patient?
   a. It delivers more oxygen than an Ambu bag
   b. It is the only way to deliver 100 percent oxygen
   c. It protects the airway from aspiration
   d. It carries the same advantages as the bag-valve mask delivery system

Answer: c. The ET tube has a cuff that protects the airway from any aspiration of stomach contents that could occur with vomiting.

4. What is the main reason why it is a good idea to intubate the head-injury patient?

a. They tend to have a decreased drive to breathe

b. They may also have maxillofacial trauma requiring intubation

c. They may have increased intracranial pressure and need hyperventilation

d. They tend to become unconscious over time so intubation early is important

Answer: c. These patients are developing increased intracranial pressure, especially if they have a bleed or a significant contusion in the brain. Intubating them and hyperventilating them can prevent hypercarbia and can reduce the risks of brain herniation syndrome.

5. What is the most important thing to do when intubating a patient with head and neck trauma?

a. Use the smallest ET tube size possible because there will be swelling.

b. Visualize the vocal cords when intubating the patient.

c. Use the largest ET tube size possible in order to keep the airway open.

d. Do not attempt to intubate and go straight to doing a cricothyrotomy.

Answer: b. The anatomy may be disrupted so the key thing in intubation is to make no assumptions about the placement of the vocal cords and attempt to visualize them directly while doing the procedure.

6. In evaluating the trauma patient's ventilation status, what can you suspect if the patient is agitated?

a. Hypovolemia

b. Hypercarbia

c. Hypoxia

d. Upper airway obstruction

Answer: c. An agitated patient suggests hypoxia, which can be confirmed by an oxygen saturation level. These patients need a definitive airway and should have ventilatory support with high flow oxygen by whatever means is most appropriate for the patient's condition.

7. Which of the following airway management techniques involves providing a definitive airway in a trauma patient?

a. Laryngeal mask airway

b. Laryngeal tube airway

c. Endotracheal intubation

d. All of the above

Answer: c. The only definitive airway listed is the placement of an endotracheal tube. The LMA and the LTA are both temporary measures and do not represent a definitive airway. Eventually, an ET tube must be placed instead.

8. At what Glasgow Coma Score or below should the trauma patient be intubated and ventilated using high glow oxygen?

a. Ten

b. Eight

c. Six

d. Four

Answer: b. At a Glasgow Coma Score of eight or less, the trauma patient should be intubated and ventilated.

9. What finding would be a relative contraindication to having a nasotracheal tube placed?
    a. Battle's sign
    b. Raccoon's eyes
    c. CSF from the nose
    d. All of the above

Answer: d. Any of the above signs indicate a possible basilar skull fracture, which would be a relative contraindication to having a nasotracheal tube placed.

10. How much of a bolus of warmed lactated Ringer's solution should be given to an adult trauma patient in shock?
    a. 500 cc
    b. 1-2 liters
    c. 2-3 liters
    d. 20 ml/kg

Answer: b. Adults should receive a 1-2-liter bolus of warmed isotonic fluid as part of the initial resuscitation of shock. Children should receive 20 ml/kg IV fluid.

Chapter 11: ATLS for Children and Infants

In the previous chapter, we focused on basic Advanced Trauma Life Support protocols for the trauma patient, emphasizing airway management, ventilation, and the treatment of shock. Much of the information provided related directly to adults with trauma. In this chapter, the main focus will be on the trauma support of infants and children as they present unique challenges in the management of trauma patients.

Pediatric Trauma Overview

Trauma is the greatest cause of morbidity and mortality in children living in the United States. Because children are not simply small adults, they need a unique approach to their injuries and attention to the details that will make or break a successful resuscitation in the injured child. Unfortunately, there are only about eighty accredited pediatric trauma hospitals in the US, making the care of pediatric trauma patients something that is normally not done by a well-trained healthcare team.

Some type of trauma is the leading cause of death in children over the age of one year. Injuries and subsequent death causes more deaths in children than any other cause of childhood death combined. Unintentional injury causes about sixty-five percent of all injury deaths in kids under the age of 19 years. This means that thirty-five percent of the time, the cause of traumatic death is intentional, such as from suicide, or homicide. About 20,000 children and teens die from injury with forty times that number being hospitalized for injury and more than a thousand times that number being seen and treated in the emergency department. About 50,000 children suffer from some type of permanent disability from being injured, with closed head injury being the most common cause of this type of disability.

There are certain factors that influence whether or not a child is injured. Gender and age have a lot to do with the epidemiology of injuries in children. Males under the age of eighteen years have more injuries and deaths from injuries when compared to females. In infants and toddlers, the most common cause of an injury is a fall, while in school-age kids and teens, bicycle accidents are the most common cause of injuries. Helmet use has resulted in improved outcomes among this age group.

About thirty-five percent of the time, the childhood injury happens within the home in familiar surroundings, pointing to a strong need for parents and other loved ones to support the child by child-proofing all homes in which infants, toddlers, and preschoolers live.

The largest majority of pediatric injuries happen as a result of some type of blunt trauma, with penetrating injuries accounting for about 10-20 percent of hospital admissions among children. Among penetrating injuries, it is gunshot wounds that cause the majority of these injuries, with things like metal pieces off of cars and shrapnel injuries accounting for a smaller proportion of pediatric penetrating traumatic injuries.

Interestingly, burn injuries tend to be seen in children about one to four years of age, while upper extremity fractures were found to be more common among kids aged five to nine years. Adolescents tend to dominate, when it comes to traumatic brain injuries and lower extremity fractures.

Head Injuries

Head injuries represent the most common isolated injures in children and is the leading cause of death from injury in children. The children that do survive, however, recover faster and to a greater degree when compared to adults. Children have somewhat of a reserve system going on in the CNS that allow the child to recover well, even when parts of the brain are seriously injured.

Unfortunately, among toddlers less than two years of age, physical abuse by an adult is the most common cause of a head injury. The biggest problem in this age group is called "shaken baby syndrome" or SBS, which happens when an adult strongly shakes a baby, resulting in the brain hitting up against the interior of the skull. These children not only have contusions of the brain but they have subarachnoid hemorrhages, subdural hemorrhages, and retinal bleeding as major findings. In kids older than this, falls and accidents related to a vehicle (bicycle, motor vehicle, or pedestrian accident) predominate.

Brain injuries in children tend to cause diffuse swelling more so than a hematoma or other space-occupying condition. This means that, early in the evaluation of a head trauma patient's head injury, the CT scan may be negative. MRI scanning is superior because it shows the obscuration of the white and gray matter border that is typical of cerebral edema. These children need treatment for increased intracranial pressure, such as hyperventilation and mannitol.

The Glasgow Coma Scale (GCS) is used primarily for the determination of the status of the child with a closed head injury. The score ranges from 3 to 15, with higher numbers reflecting a better CNS status. Even with relatively normal or high scores on the GCS, a CT scan or MRI scan should be done if there is an ongoing altered level of consciousness or a history of unconsciousness that lasted longer than five minutes after the injury.

Unfortunately, children who present with a unilateral dilated pupil, a GCS score of less than eight or a penetrating gunshot wound to the head have a high mortality rate at up to 98 percent. A major cause of morbidity in those children who survive is not providing an adequately aggressive resuscitation that avoids hypoxia and hypotension, which cause prolonged CNS injury.

The metabolic demand is elevated in children with head injuries that can cause secondary problems, such as fever and seizures because the child's brain needs a high level of nutritional support that is sometimes not given. This points to a strong need to provide top-notch nutritional support to children injured with CNS trauma as soon as the child is somewhat stabilized. Ideally, the nutritional support should be enteral rather than parenteral so the child who cannot eat on his or her own should have a feeding tube.

A mild head injury is referred to as a concussion. It is the mildest form of head injury, which may or may not have a loss of consciousness associated with it. The GCS is between fourteen and fifteen and, if there is loss of consciousness, it is brief and the child only has mild amnesia surrounding the event itself. These children can simply be observed and discharged after a six-hour observation period. These children can have mild CNS dysfunction and other symptoms after their injury but they usually resolve within three months of the injury.

Children with a mild head injury probably don't need to be exposed to the radiation they would get from a head CT and only about five percent of these kids will have any positive findings on CT scan of the head.

The very young child with a head injury will be difficult to evaluate because they don't talk and cannot indicate their symptoms. There is a higher rate of skull fractures in this age group, however, so a CT scan may need to be done to evaluate the child for a basilar skull fracture or other skull fracture. If the child was unconscious for more than a minute, have multiple vomiting episodes, have a bulging fontanel, or have any focal neurologic findings, a CT scan should be done. In the absence of these things, a plain film can be done (with a CT scan performed if the plain film reveals a skull fracture).

In a severe pediatric head injury, the goal is to maximize the delivery of oxygen and perfusion of the brain after the injury as these things can prevent secondary injury to the brain. Intracranial pressure monitoring (ICP monitoring) should be done in any child with a GCS score of 8 or less as the cerebral edema can cause an increased ICP. Only about two percent of kids will have an epidural hematoma and most of the rest of children don't have any space-occupying lesion that would show up on CT scan.

The finding of increased intracranial pressure can still be there if the child has open sutures, which partially accommodate for the increase in brain swelling but not enough to justify not checking the ICP on these children as well. Children can benefit from a ventriculostomy catheter, which will both drain off excess fluid and can monitor the ICP. A Camino monitor will detect the ICP but won't drain fluid off, which makes the ventriculostomy catheter superior.

If the ICP becomes elevated, the treatment of choice is to drain off any excess ventricular fluid, sedate the child, give IV mannitol, give hypertonic saline, and perform a neuromuscular blockade. There is no need to use hyperventilation in this age group because it tends not to work and has a lot of side effects that can injure the brain. A second-line treatment if the first-line treatments are ineffective includes hypothermia treatments, which work on younger children the best. A decompressive craniectomy is reserved for very severe cases of increased ICP that doesn't respond to other measures.

Spinal Cord Injuries in Children

Because of the flexibility of children's necks, the finding of a cervical spine injury isn't very common in children. Even so, an injured child with the potential for a C-spine injury should be immobilized and imaged to make sure there is no spinal cord injury. About 40 percent of spinal cord injuries in children come from car accidents with fractures mostly of the first two vertebrae. If these aren't detected and treated, the neurological outcome is generally very poor.

About ten to twenty percent of kids will have a spinal cord injury that doesn't show up on imaging studies. This is because the spinal cord or the spinal nerve roots get stretched and deformed but there will be no severing of the cord. These children, fortunately, will have transient severe symptoms that resolve within hours of the injury. Children with transient paralysis after an injury to the spine should be closely evaluated because any re-injury to the area can result in a permanent deficit. Sometimes, an MRI evaluation will show something not seen on plain films or CT scan of the spine.

Neck Injuries in Children

Children with neck injuries have a high incidence of airway problems so the airway must be secured soon after seeing the child. They can have expanding hematomas, bleeding, or soft tissue swelling that can adversely affect the airway. In less common circumstances, the esophagus can be ruptured or otherwise injured in a neck injury.

Oropharyngeal injuries in kids usually happen as a result of a fall. Because these areas are highly vascular, there can be a great deal of bleeding and bruising, even from a relatively minor injury. Any laceration of the tongue or lip can be repaired with absorbable sutures that won't have to be removed at any time after the injury and will provide the best cosmesis, especially if plastic surgery techniques are used to carefully suture lacerations of these areas. Mild lacerations of the tongue do not have to be treated; however, deep lacerations will cause a deformity of the tongue if not repaired using absorbable sutures.

Any injuries involving the teeth or alveolar bone should be referred to a dentist for full evaluation to include x-rays and repair of missing or broken teeth. Injuries to the parotid gland area are at a high risk for cranial nerve VII injuries, so they must be carefully evaluated and referred for treatment by a head and neck surgeon if a cranial nerve injury is suspected.

Eye Trauma in Children

Eye injuries in children tend to occur in sporting activities. Eye trauma in kids can cause significant deficits in vision, in part because the eye is still developing up to the age of nine years. Most eye traumas are mild, such as corneal abrasions or conjunctival hemorrhages. In the situation of a more serious injury, such as a ruptured globe, nothing should be done except for covering the eye and referring the injury to a qualified ophthalmologist. All eye injuries should have an assessment of the vision as any injury to the eye can affect the child's eyesight.

Eyelid lacerations need to be carefully managed—not only for cosmetic reasons but for the reason that the lacrimal duct can become injured and needs microscopic repair by an ophthalmologist. Fractures of the face involving the maxillary sinus can result in double vision because of entrapment of the extraocular muscles of the eye. Symptoms of eye pain or foreign body sensation without any obvious findings on exam indicate the need for a fluorescein stain examination in order to rule out a corneal abrasion or small corneal foreign body.

Thoracic Injuries in Children

Chest trauma makes up the second highest cause of death in childhood trauma and accounts for about five percent of hospitalized children who have trauma. Most injuries are blunt trauma injuries from motor vehicle accidents and are usually associated with multisystem trauma. It takes a greater insult to cause a pediatric thoracic injury when compared to an adult thoracic injury because the child has more compliance of the chest wall than is seen in adults. Things like bruising of lung tissue and pneumothorax can be seen in the absence of any rib fractures or external signs of trauma. Penetrating injuries tend to cause both pneumothorax and hemothorax—both of which generally need surgical intervention.

If the chest cavity is tapped and at least twenty percent of the child's blood volume is extracted, the child needs an urgent chest exploration because there is a high incidence of intercostal artery bleeding behind this kind of scenario. A chest CT can usually identify this injury, which can be present even if the plain chest x-ray is negative. A pulse oximetry reading can identify those children with severe chest injuries when the physical examination and plain films show nothing.

Children have a high incidence of pulmonary contusions with severe chest trauma. The major complication is edema and inflammation of the lung parenchyma, which leads to atelectasis, swelling of lung tissue, and lung consolidation, all of which can cause secondary tachypnea and hypoxemia. The chest x-ray may be normal initially but will show the contusion in up to seventy percent of cases. These can be treated with rest and oxygen, with most children recovering within a week to ten days after the injury.

Traumatic rupture of the diaphragm can occur but it only occurs in about one percent of children with a blunt traumatic injury to the chest. The left diaphragm is affected more often than the right. The diagnosis can be made by passing a nasogastric tube down to the stomach and taking a chest x-ray. If the tip of the NG tube is in the thorax, a diaphragm rupture can be assumed. This generally needs surgical repair because the stomach contents and the rest of the abdominal viscera can travel up through the diaphragm, impinging motion of the lungs.

Abdominal Injuries in Children

There are anatomical differences in the abdomens of children that make them have a greater incidence of abdominal trauma, even in situations where the trauma seems minor. They have undeveloped musculature in the abdomen so that it provides little protection against forces that might be generated in a motor vehicle accident or fall.

Most childhood abdominal trauma is blunt trauma rather than penetrating trauma. They are especially vulnerable to solid organ trauma, with the spleen being the most likely organ to be damaged in a blunt trauma injury, followed by the liver and kidneys. The death rate for blunt trauma injuries in children is higher than the mortality rate in penetrating trauma because many of these children will also have CNS and thoracic trauma (because their bodies are so small).

Whenever blunt trauma has occurred to a child, the question of how to work these up comes up. CT scans are effective but give the child unnecessary radiation. A better test is the FAST exam, which stands for "focused abdominal sonography for trauma". This test is a bit of a misnomer because it can also be used in thoracic injuries. It is a quick ultrasound of the abdomen and chest that can effectively pick up free air in the abdomen, blood in the abdomen, thoracic blood, pericardial blood, or obvious injury to the solid organs of the abdomen. It can miss a solid organ injury so, if the exam is negative and there is still a high index of suspicion for an abdominal solid organ injury, a CT scan of the abdomen is necessary.

A CT scan of the abdomen is a good test if there is obvious bruising of the abdominal wall and gross hematuria as it can detect kidney injuries that might not show up on a FAST examination. Unfortunately, the CT scan does not easily show up a hollow viscus rupture, while the FAST examination is good for this. Up to a third of all kids with a solid viscus injury and free air in the abdomen will have a normal CT scan of the abdomen but will have findings at the time of surgery or through a FAST examination.

The diagnostic peritoneal lavage or DPL is not done often on children because the CT scan is better at identifying the exact location of the bleeding than can be gotten by a DPL examination. A DPL is only indicated when a child needs immediate surgery and there is no time to do a CT scan. DPL examinations are fast and, if negative, can effectively rule out a solid organ injury. In situations where a solid organ injury is suspected, the CT scan is superior to the FAST examination because up to forty percent of minor liver and spleen injuries will not be picked up by a FAST examination. As many as 11 percent of severe liver and spleen injuries can be missed by a FAST examination.

The finding of abdominal wall bruising on clinical examination after a significant blunt trauma injury should raise the clinical suspicion that a serious injury is present in the abdomen. The child should have a FAST examination or CT scan of the abdomen. If a CT scan shows free fluid and no solid organ injury, a ruptured viscus is a highly likely injury. Vertebral fractures occur to a high degree in children who have a positive "seatbelt sign"—which is bruising of the abdomen where the seatbelt restrained the child.

There are more blunt trauma injuries to the stomach after an accident than is seen in adults. The injury is usually a blow-out injury secondary to pressure on the stomach by an external force. The stomach is not well protected by the rib cage in children so it can easily be injured. Blood in the nasogastric tube after its insertion should greatly increase the suspicion for this type of injury.

The most common injury in restrained children who are involved in a motor vehicle accident is a ruptured viscus. The rapid deceleration against the seatbelt causes compression of the abdomen at that level, forcing the anterior abdominal wall to push in toward the spine. This increases the intra-abdominal pressure so that any hollow organ can be easily torn or ruptured.

If the viscus doesn't rupture completely, it can easily bruise, causing a large hematoma that can obstruct the intestinal lumen. This type of obstruction can show up weeks after the initial injury.

Up to half of all children with intra-abdominal injuries secondary to blunt force trauma will have some type of retroperitoneal injury. This can be an injury to the kidneys or to the spine. Flexion-distraction lumbar spinal injuries are common complications of being restrained and having blunt force placed upon the abdomen by the seat belt.

Fewer than half of all children with an obvious small intestinal perforation will show peritoneal signs or peritonitis when first examined. They may have abdominal tenderness as the first finding, with fever, rebound tenderness, and a rigid abdomen happening hours or a day later. If, on surgical evaluation, more than 50 percent of the diameter of the lumen is obstructed, the area must be resected. If, on the other hand, less than half of the luminal wall diameter is ruptured, the tear can be repaired primarily without removing any of the viscus.

Most isolated rectal injuries are secondary to sexual abuse of the child. This area is extremely sensitive so, if there is an examination to be undertaken, it should be done under general anesthesia to protect the child from the pain of this type of exam. Tears of the rectal mucosa or anus can usually be watched and will heal primarily without surgical intervention. If the internal anal sphincter is involved, however, surgery to repair it may be necessary.

If a child is clinically stable and has a solid organ injury, they can be monitored with serial ultrasounds and clinical evaluation of their overall status without having to resort to reparative surgery. Most of the time, the bleeding will slow and stop, with secondary healing of the solid organ. It is estimated that simply watching the stable child will later result in having to do surgery about five percent of the time. This makes observation of the vast majority of solid organ injuries a viable option. If multiple solid organs are injured, the rate of having to do surgery goes up and non-operative care is less likely to be successful.

As mentioned, spleen injuries are the most common solid organ injury seen in children with blunt trauma. Because these children risk having serious infections if their spleen is removed, the primary goal is to try to preserve the spleen and this means simply observing the injury if the child is hemodynamically stable. Most of the time, the spleen will stop bleeding on its own and will heal without any significant intervention. The child will need ICU evaluation and monitoring for 48 hours after the injury is detected to make sure they remain stable.

Liver injuries behave much like splenic injuries in that they tend to stop bleeding on their own as long as none of the major veins are disrupted. These children can be watched without doing any type of interventional surgery and about 90 percent of them will not need surgery at a later time. The only exception to this is the major liver injury in a child who is not hemodynamically stable. Delayed bleeding will happen in up to three percent of cases with a death rate of 18 percent. Having surgery on standby and observing stable patients, however, will be successfully managed without intervention in the vast majority of cases.

Pancreatic injuries can happen secondary to a blunt trauma to the abdomen. A typical mechanism of action of these types of injuries is when a child falls off his or her bicycle and strikes the handlebars with their upper abdomen. CT scanning is necessary to evaluate these injuries but the ability to pick up a rupture of the pancreatic duct is difficult with just a CT scan. ERCP (Endoscopic retrograde pancreatography) may be necessary to evaluate the collecting system of the pancreas and bile ducts. An elevation in amylase and lipase levels point strongly to a pancreatic injury that will need to be further evaluated. If the pancreas is severely injured, part of it may have to be removed.

Kidney injuries can also happen with blunt abdominal trauma in about 10-20 percent of cases. The kidneys in children tend to be less well protected than the kidneys in adults because they have less perirenal fat to cushion them. A blow to the back or flank area can also cause a renal injury, although this is less common than an abdominal injury. Like other solid organ injuries, kidney injuries can be monitored as long as the patient is stable and no surgical intervention needs to take place unless the injury is very severe or the child is hemodynamically unstable. If there is an expanding hematoma, especially one that is pulsatile, the injury can be assumed to be severe and surgery is indicated to repair or remove the kidney.

Orthopedic Injuries in Children

About a third of all children seen for trauma will have at least one skeletal fracture. This means that a careful evaluation of all of the child's extremities should take place, checking for tenderness or deformities seen in in a fracture setting. Distal pulses and neurological status need to be assessed any time there is a fracture as any break in the bone can damage nearby nerves or blood vessels. To that end, pulses and nerve function should be assessed in every extremity of a child trauma victim. Along with extremity fractures, children have a high rate of skull fractures and vertebral fractures, especially if they have been multiply injured in a serious accident or fall.

Key Takeaways

- Children have unique patterns of injury and are not simply small adults.
- Head injuries are the leading cause of morbidity and mortality among injured children.
- Children have fewer isolated injuries and are more likely to have injuries spanning many body areas, such as both the thorax and the abdomen.
- Many solid organ injuries in children can simply be monitored without surgery as only a small percentage of the time will a later surgery be necessary because of failure to heal spontaneously.

Quiz

1. What percentage of childhood injuries and death stem from an accidental or non-intentional injury?
    a. Thirty-five percent
    b. Fifty percent
    c. Sixty-five percent
    d. Eighty percent

Answer: c. About sixty-five percent of childhood injuries and death are secondary to a non-intentional injury, with the rest being the result of suicide or homicide.

2. What is the most common cause of childhood disability secondary to an injury?
    a. Blunt abdominal trauma
    b. Orthopedic injuries
    c. Pelvic fractures
    d. Head injuries

Answer: d. The vast majority of injury-related disabilities in childhood stem from the after-effects of head injuries.

3. What is the most common cause of injuries in children under the age of three years?
    a. Motor vehicle accidents
    b. Falls
    c. Bicycle injuries
    d. Non-accidental injuries

Answer: b. Falls account for the major cause of injuries in infants and children under the age of three years.

4. What is the most common cause of closed head trauma in a child under the age of two years?
    a. Motor vehicle accident
    b. Fall from a height
    c. Pedestrian accident
    d. Shaken baby syndrome

Answer: d. Among children under the age of two years, shaken baby syndrome is perhaps the most common cause of closed head trauma, resulting in a variety of different brain insults.

5. Why is magnetic resonance imaging (MRI scan) better than a CT scan when evaluating a child having a closed head injury?
    a. It can pick up cerebral edema better than a CT scan.
    b. It can show focal areas of bleeding better than a CT scan.

c. It can show increased intracranial pressure better than a CT scan.

d. It can show contra-coupe injuries better than a CT scan.

Answer: a. An MRI is superior to a CT scan when evaluating a child with a closed head injury because it picks up cerebral edema better and many children have only cerebral edema as a result of their head injury rather than major bleeds or other focal findings.

6. Why is a feeding tube so important to treating CNS injuries in children?

a. Children who lose weight after a CNS injury have a worsened prognosis than those who don't lose weight.

b. The child's high metabolic demands after a CNS injury can cause secondary brain injury if not fed early in the course of the recovery.

c. These children need to eat but are at a high risk of aspiration so they should be fed via a feeding tube.

d. Most children with a head injury are on a ventilator so they need either enteral or parenteral feeding.

Answer: b. The child with a CNS injury has an increased metabolic demand so they need to have enteral feeding to avoid starving the brain of nutrients as it heals from an injury.

7. What spinal cord injury would be most common in a child after a motor vehicle accident?

a. C1 or C2

b. C6 or C7

c. Any thoracic vertebral injury

d. L3 to L5

Answer: a. The most common spinal cord injury in a child after a motor vehicle accident is a C1 or C2 injury, both of which can result in serious neurological sequelae if injured and not quickly managed.

8. In treating a child with a neck injury, what must be a top priority in evaluating and managing the injury?

a. They have a high incidence of upper esophageal rupture.

b. They have a high incidence of lower cervical spine injuries when the neck is injured.

c. They have narrow airway passages that can easily get compromised when the neck is injured.

d. They tend to have a high incidence of cranial nerve injuries with neck injuries.

Answer: c. The airway is the biggest issue with pediatric neck injuries. They have a narrow airway that can easily become compromised because of hematomas or swelling of the neck after an injury to the area.

9. What injury is likely if a child sustains a chest wall injury and has a greater than twenty percent of their total blood volume in a chest tube evacuation of a hemothorax?

a. Jugular vein rupture

b. Thoracic aortic rupture

c. Subclavian vein rupture

d. Intercostal artery disruption

Answer: d. A common injury resulting in a large hemothorax in children is an intercostal artery rupture, which needs surgical exploration and repair in order to manage the bleeding, which tends to be profuse.

10. What is the primary rational behind simply observing stable splenic injuries in children?

   a. The child has a high mortality rate during this type of surgical intervention so it is avoided at all costs.

   b. The child risks overwhelming infections for the rest of his or her life without a spleen so it should be preserved if possible.

   c. The rate of dying from surgery to remove the spleen is higher than the rate of dying from a ruptured spleen that isn't treated.

   d. If the child is stable with this type of injury, only about 35 percent need to have surgery to remove the spleen later so it is preserved if possible.

Answer: b. The child without a spleen risks overwhelming infections for the rest of his or her life without a spleen so, if the child is stable, the spleen should be observed and preserved if possible.

Summary

This course was intended to offer a broad base of information to the potential healthcare provider of the basics of Basic Life Support, Advanced Cardiac Life Support, and Advanced Trauma Life Support. Nearly every healthcare provider will face having to care for the critically-ill or critically-injured patient and will need to know how best to stabilize these types of patients so they can receive definitive care.

The first chapter involved a thorough discussion of the assessment of the unconscious patient. These patients represent a unique challenge to the healthcare provider as they cannot verbally relay any symptoms and most are seriously ill, requiring urgent evaluation and management.

In chapter two, we had a discussion of Basic Life Support for Adults. While Basic Life Support is intended to be used by anyone, there are unique aspects to the provision of this type of vital patient care that are different when a skilled healthcare provider delivers the service as opposed to a lay person.

The third chapter of the course involved the Basic Life Support protocols for infants and children. Infants and children have cardiac arrests for different reasons than in adults but still require CPR during an arrest situation. The protocols to be followed by the lay person and healthcare provider alike were a part of this chapter.

In chapter four, the focus of the discussion was on how the automated external defibrillator works and how it is best put into use in the field. You saw how the AED has the potential to save many lives because it quickly restores the rhythm of an adult or child with a non-survivable rhythm strip.

Chapter five of the course was an introduction into the rhythms seen in Advanced Cardiac Life Support. Each rhythm has unique features that can be identified by the healthcare provider, setting the pace for intervention by the ACLS team.

The algorithms used in the adult patient with an abnormal rhythm or who is in a cardiac arrest situation were the focus of the sixth chapter of the course. Each rhythm and clinical situation has a specific algorithm to follow. The intricacies of these algorithms were covered in that chapter as they apply to real-world situations.

The seventh chapter of the course was a discussion of the medications used in cardiac arrest situations and in treating arrhythmias. The purposes and dosages of the medications were covered as part of understanding how they are put into use in various arrhythmia and arrest situations.

The eighth chapter of the course introduced pediatric advanced life support or PALS. Children have different common rhythm disturbances and suffer from arrests for very different reasons than adults and require a different approach than is seen in adults who have an arrest situation.

In the ninth chapter of the course, prehospital trauma assessment and management were discussed. The prehospital rescuer is in a special situation of being able to have a positive impact on the survival of the critically-injured patient.

The tenth chapter of the course was a discussion of Advanced Trauma Life Support or ATLS for adults. Trauma patients can have a variety of injuries and often require intense resuscitation soon after being injured if they are to survive.

The eleventh chapter of the course discussed the trauma situations seen in pediatric patients. Pediatric patients are highly likely to be multiply traumatized in an accident or fall and usually require evaluation and treatment of more than one body area after they become injured.

Course Questions & Answers

1. In evaluating an unconscious patient, what places their situation beyond the scope of management of treating just the unconscious state?
   a. Lack of ability to respond to pain
   b. Decorticate posturing
   c. Absence of a pulse
   d. Irregular breathing

Answer: c. A patient who does not have a pulse has cardiorespiratory arrest and this is far beyond that which is found simply by being unconscious.

2. What question asked by a person with an altered mental status is most likely to be answered incorrectly with mild mental status changes?
   a. What is your name?
   b. What is your birthdate?
   c. Where do you live?
   d. What day is it?

Answer: d. Patients with an altered mental status will have a loss of orientation to time and place first before they will have a loss of memory of their name, birthdate, and address, which are stored in long-term memory and are more easily retained by the patient, even when they have significant mental status changes.

3. What is not one of the top three things to be assessed in a patient who is unconscious?
   a. Pupillary light reflex
   b. Presence of an adequate airway
   c. Presence of spontaneous respirations
   d. Adequacy of pulse

Answer: a. The first three things than need to be assessed in a patient who is unconscious include their airway, presence of spontaneous respirations, and adequacy of the pulse. Any assessment of their neurological status should be secondary to those three things.

4. You believe a person has fainted but you have no history as to the patient's overall state of health. You believe the patient is male and about 30 years of age. When do you consider calling 911 for the syncopal episode?
   a. As soon as the person has fainted.
   b. The patient has a seizure after fainting.
   c. The patient has not regained consciousness after five minutes.
   d. The patient has not regained consciousness after ten minutes.

Answer: b. Anytime a patient has a seizure as part of their syncopal episode, 911 should be called. This is especially true if you have no history as to whether or not the patient has a

98

known seizure disorder. In the absence of a seizure, it is safe to wait at least one minute before considering calling 911 as most patients with a simple syncopal episode will regain consciousness within a minute. Waiting longer than a minute is not advised.

5. What assessment is not a part of the Glasgow Coma Scale?
    a. Pupillary light reflex
    b. Eye opening
    c. Verbal response
    d. Motor response

Answer: a. The three things assessed in a GCS include eye opening, verbal response, and motor response. The pupillary light reflex is often assessed in comatose patients but is not a part of the GCS assessment.

6. The patient you are evaluating is moaning but not saying any words. What GCS rating would you give the patient?
    a. One
    b. Two
    c. Three
    d. Four

Answer: b. The patient who moans only is incomprehensible, meaning they have a GCS score for verbal response of just two.

7. Which blood test should be done first in evaluating a patient with unconsciousness as this is crucial in the first steps taken?
    a. Potassium
    b. Glucose
    c. Troponin
    d. ABGs

Answer: b. A glucose level should be done using a glucometer, which can be done at the scene. The other testing needs hospital equipment to do and should be done after a blood sugar evaluation.

8. What antidote should be given to all unconscious patients without a history but who are without evidence of trauma?
    a. Naloxone
    b. Hyperbaric oxygen
    c. Acetyl cysteine
    d. Activated charcoal

Answer: a. Naloxone is the antidote for an opiate ingestion-related state of unconsciousness. It should be given anytime the patient has no history but is believed not to have suffered trauma as opiate ingestion can be fatal within a few minutes.

9. Which diagnostic or imaging test should be done first after getting the patient to a hospital or an emergency department in an unconscious patient?
   a. Chest x-ray
   b. CT scan of the head
   c. Electrocardiogram
   d. Flat plate of the abdomen

Answer: c. Diagnostically, the first test that should be done upon reaching a hospital or emergency department is the EKG as this will test for any MI or arrhythmia that could require urgent treatment in the unconscious patient.

10. The patient is unconscious and has a pulse that is weak and thready. Their skin is red and they have facial swelling and hives. You do not have a history. What urgent treatment can you give them?
    a. D50W
    b. Epinephrine IV
    c. Naloxone IV
    d. Oral or rectal glucagon

Answer: b. The clinical abrasion is suggestive of anaphylaxis, which involves giving IV epinephrine ASAP, shortly after the primary survey has been completed as epinephrine can be quickly given and will resolve the unconsciousness quickly.

11. What is a cause of unconsciousness that often persists for several hours before ultimately leading to the patient's demise?
    a. Airway obstruction
    b. Anaphylaxis
    c. Hypoglycemia
    d. Septicemia

Answer: d. Most of the above symptom can kill the patient in a very short period of time, except for septicemia, which takes several hours before it has the potential to kill the patient.

12. Which surface would be the most effective surface to have the patient on for doing CPR?
    a. A hard table
    b. A firm bed
    c. The floor
    d. A cushioned couch

Answer: c. The patient would do best on the floor because they are on a hard surface and it places the CPR provider much above the victim for the best application of chest compressions.

13. What endpoint is not considered an endpoint for the provision of CPR?
    a. The provider becomes exhausted.

b. The patient has clearly died despite compressions and ventilations.

c. The patient resumes spontaneous respirations and a pulse.

d. An external defibrillation is successful.

Answer: b. All of the above are appropriate endpoints for the provision of CPR except for believing that the patient is dead. All out-of-hospital cardiac arrests should continue until a healthcare provider has decided the efforts are futile.

14. At what rate are compressions done in basic CPR?

a. Sixty beats per minute

b. Eighty beats per minute

c. A hundred beats per minute

d. One hundred twenty beats per minute

Answer: c. Compressions in CPR should be done at a rate comparable to what a normal heart rate should be under stress, which is about a hundred beats per minute.

15. About how much should the sternum be displaced during chest compressions on an adult victim?

a. One inch

b. Two inches

c. Three inches

d. Four inches

Answer: b. The sternum should be compressed at least two inches in an adult cardiac arrest patient in order for the compressions to be effective.

16. CPR is done in cycles. About how long is the cardiac compression part of a single cycle of CPR?

a. Ten compressions

b. Fifteen compressions

c. Twenty compressions

d. Thirty compressions

Answer: d. The cardiac compression phase of a single cycle of CPR begins with thirty compressions before working on ventilations. This cycle repeats itself until the patient recovers or until the provider fatigues.

17. There is a difference in the ventilatory rate when two providers are available for CPR. What is the ventilatory rate for two-provider CPR in the field?

a. Six to eight breaths a minute

b. Eight to ten breaths a minute

c. Ten to twelve breaths a minute

d. Fourteen to sixteen breaths a minute

Answer: b. With two persons available for CPR, the ventilatory rate should be about eight to ten breaths a minute.

18. What is the approximate survival rate of the average out of hospital cardiac arrest?
    a. Two percent
    b. Five percent
    c. Seven percent
    d. Ten percent

Answer: d. The average overall survival rate of an out-of-hospital arrest is about 10 percent, with about an 8 percent survival rate with a good neurological outcome.

19. What percent of witnessed cardiac arrest patients survive if their arrest is out of hospital?
    a. Ten percent
    b. Thirty-three percent
    c. Fifty percent
    d. Seventy-five percent

Answer: b. About a third or thirty-three percent of all witnessed cardiac arrests, even those out of hospital, will survive.

20. In which clinical situation should CPR be considered to be withheld?
    a. A patient with a severe traumatic injury who appears dead.
    b. A patient who is 80 years of age.
    c. A drowning patient who is obviously hypothermic.
    d. A lightning strike victim.

Answer: a. The only time CPR should be considered to be withheld is when the victim is a trauma victim who has sustained severe blunt or penetrating injury and has a low chance of survival or if a patient has a clear DNR order.

21. In which setting would gastric insufflation not be a likely problem?
    a. Mouth-to-mouth resuscitation
    b. Bag-valve-mask resuscitation
    c. Endotracheal tube resuscitation
    d. Cricothyrotomy resuscitation

Answer: c. In endotracheal tube resuscitation, there is an isolation of the airway from the GI tract, so there is no chance of gastric insufflation. The other choices do have a risk of gastric insufflation.

22. What percentage of children, on average, receive CPR if they have a cardiac arrest outside of a hospital?
    a. Ten percent

b. Thirty-three percent

c. Sixty-seven percent

d. Ninety percent

Answer: b. The sad fact is that only about thirty-three percent of patients under the age of 18 actually receive CPR after suffering an out-of-hospital cardiac arrest.

23. What is not considered a reason why giving compressions only is as successful in giving CPR to children as is giving chest compressions and ventilatory support?

a. There is enough oxygen in the lungs to exchange with carbon dioxide in the lungs for up to fifteen minutes after the arrest.

b. Gasping happens with CPR, which facilitates gas exchange.

c. Chest recoil allows for air to enter the lungs, adding to oxygenation.

d. Oxygen is forced into the chest during the compression phase.

Answer: d. Oxygen is not forced into the lungs during the compression phase, so this is not a reason why chest compressions alone is just as successful as giving compressions plus ventilatory support in children. The others are considered reasons why this is the case.

24. What mnemonic best describes the delivery of CPR to a child who has suffered an out-of-hospital cardiac arrest?

a. CAB

b. ABC

c. BAC

d. CBA

Answer: a. The mnemonic CAB stands for compressions-airway-breathing, which is the order in which tasks should happen upon caring for a child with an out-of-hospital cardiac arrest under ideal circumstances.

25. What is the recommended rate of doing compressions in a child when CPR is initiated?

a. Sixty compressions per minute

b. Eighty to one hundred compressions per minute

c. One hundred to one hundred twenty compressions per minute

d. One hundred twenty to one hundred forty compressions per minute

Answer: c. Ideally, compressions should commence at one hundred to one hundred twenty compressions per minute in a child of any age.

26. At what heart rate should chest compressions be initiated in children?

a. Zero beats per minute

b. Less than sixty beats per minute

c. Less than thirty beats per minute

d. Less than eighty beats per minute

Answer: b. If the pulse is less than sixty beats per minute in a child, chest compressions should commence because a pulse less than sixty is probably under-perfusing the child's CNS.

27. What is the cardiac cycle like for CPR in children with two rescuers?
    a. Fifteen compressions followed by two breaths
    b. Fifteen compressions followed by one breath
    c. Thirty compressions followed by two breaths
    d. Thirty compressions followed by one breath

Answer: a. The cardiac cycle for two-rescuer CPR in children is fifteen compressions followed by two breaths.

28. What is the depth of compressions to be done when CPR is performed on infants?
    a. Four cm
    b. Five cm
    c. Six cm
    d. Seven cm

Answer: a. The appropriate depth of compressions in infants is about a third of the AP diameter of their chest or about four centimeters.

29. Where should the pulse be checked for in infants undergoing CPR?
    a. Precordially
    b. Brachial artery
    c. Carotid artery
    d. Femoral artery

Answer: b. The pulse in infants should be assessed for about ten seconds at the brachial artery in infants.

30. What is considered the longest period of time between compressions in child CPR?
    a. Five seconds
    b. Thirty seconds
    c. Ten seconds
    d. There should be no interruption in CPR at all.

Answer: c. if there is a provider who can assess the pulse, there can be an interruption of up to ten seconds in order to check for a spontaneous return of a pulse in child CPR.

31. What is an acceptable respiratory rate for ventilating a child undergoing CPR?
    a. Eight breaths a minute
    b. Ten breaths a minute
    c. Fourteen breaths a minute
    d. Twenty-four breaths a minute

Answer: c. The rate of ventilations in a child undergoing CPR is about twelve to twenty breaths per minute so fourteen breaths per minute is appropriate.

32. Which is one thing that the AED cannot do?
    a. Tell when a shockable rhythm or a non-shockable rhythm is present.
    b. Identify and say what the rhythm pattern is.

c. Tell when the patient is moving.

d. Tell the user when to check for the patient's pulse.

Answer: b. The AED can do many things but it cannot say what the exact rhythm pattern actually is. It can only say if the rhythm is shockable or not shockable.

33. How specific is the AED in detecting ventricular fibrillation?

a. 50 percent

b. 75 percent

c. 90 percent

d. 100 percent

Answer: d. The AED is nearly 100 percent specific in the detection of ventricular fibrillation but is only 76-96 percent sensitive.

34. What is the main reason why most defibrillators are biphasic?

a. The time to charge to full power is shorter.

b. It is superior in defibrillating over the monophasic defibrillator.

c. Biphasic defibrillators are less dangerous to use than monophasic defibrillators.

d. Monophasic defibrillators don't deliver a strong enough charge.

Answer: a. The two main reasons why most defibrillators are biphasic are that the time to charge is less and the battery life is longer. It is not superior technically to monophasic defibrillation and is not necessarily safer than monophasic defibrillation.

35. At what response time is it considered the maximal time acceptable for the AED to be successful in improving survival rates?

a. 2-4 minutes

b. 4-6 minutes

c. 6-8 minutes

d. 8-10 minutes

Answer: b. A response rate for an AED past about 4-6 minutes is probably going to be ineffective in improving patient survival. This points highly to the advantage of having AEDs in places where an arrest is most likely to be witnessed.

36. What is the primary pacemaker in the heart when a patient has premature atrial contractions?

a. Atrioventricular node

b. Sinoatrial node

c. Atrial wall

d. Ventricular septum

Answer: b. With premature atrial contractions, the primary pacemaker is the sinoatrial node but it is stimulated to contract at a rate that is faster and out of the normal rhythm of the heart.

37. By definition, sinus tachycardia has an atrial contraction rate of at least how many beats per minute?
    a. 70 bpm
    b. 90 bpm
    c. 100 bpm
    c. 120 bpm

Answer: c. By definition, sinus tachycardia involves a sinus rhythm/atrial contraction rate of at least 100 beats per minute.   A normal sinus rhythm is between 60 and 100 bpm.

38. What is the atrial rate in atrial flutter?
    a. 300 bpm
    b. 200 bpm
    c. 150 bpm
    d. 100 bpm

Answer: a. In atrial flutter, there is a re-entrant rhythm, in which there is a cycle that runs an atrial contraction rate of about three hundred beats per minute.

39. Which is not considered a major cause of sinus bradycardia?
    a. Hyperthermia
    b. Sleep apnea
    c. Being athletic
    d. Sick sinus syndrome

Answer: a. All of the above can cause sinus bradycardia except for hyperthermia, which tends to cause sinus tachycardia instead.

40. What is the approximate heart rate in a junctional rhythm?
    a. 20-40 bpm
    b. 40-60 bpm
    c. 60-80 bpm
    d. 80-100 bpm

Answer: b. The heart rate originates in a place in the heart where the natural automaticity produces a rate of 40-60 bpm unless the rhythm is accelerated by certain drugs or medical states.

41. Where does the heart beat electrical rhythm originate in a junctional rhythm?
    a. SA node
    b. Bundle of His
    c. AV node
    d. Purkinje fibers

Answer: c. In a junctional rhythm, the AV node is the place where the rhythm originates, making a natural heart rate of about 40-60 bpm.

42. Which electrolyte abnormality is unassociated with the development of PVCs?
    a. Hypokalemia
    b. Hypercalcemia
    c. Hyponatremia
    d. Hypomagnesemia

Answer: c. All of the above electrolyte abnormalities can cause PVCs except for hyponatremia.

43. Prolapse of what valve can lead to the development of PVCs?
    a. Tricuspid
    b. Pulmonic
    c. Aortic
    d. Mitral

Answer: d. Mitral valve prolapse can cause frequent PVCs in the absence of any other heart disease.

44. What is the fastest rate that can be obtained in ventricular tachycardia?
    a. 200 bpm
    b. 250 bpm
    c. 300 bpm
    d. 350 bpm

Answer: c. The fastest ventricular tachycardia (also referred to as ventricular flutter) is about 300 beats per minute. There is very little cardiac output at this rate and urgent intervention is necessary.

45. How many abnormal QRS complexes in a row qualifies as being ventricular tachycardia?
    a. Two
    b. Three
    c. Eight
    d. Twenty

Answer: b. At least three abnormal QRS complexes suggestive of a ventricular focus must be present in order to have a diagnosis of ventricular tachycardia.

46. Of the arrhythmias a person can have, which would be considered the most life-threatening?
    a. Ventricular fibrillation
    b. Frequent premature ventricular contractions
    c. Torsades de Pointes
    d. Atrial flutter

Answer: a. With ventricular fibrillation, there is nearly no cardiac output and death is imminent without defibrillation. This is a highly life-threatening arrhythmia to have.

47. When a person has sustained wide and fast QRS complexes that differ in morphology from beat-to-beat, what is this called?
    a. Ventricular flutter
    b. Ventricular fibrillation
    c. Ventricular tachycardia
    d. Torsades de pointes

Answer: d. Torsades de pointes is a type of ventricular tachycardia in which the QRS complexes differ in morphology from beat-to-beat. It has a very characteristic ECG rhythm appearance.

48. Which electrolyte disturbance would you most likely see in a patient with acquired Torsades de pointes?
    a. Hypernatremia
    b. Hypomagnesemia
    c. Hyperkalemia
    d. Hypocalcemia

Answer: b. Low potassium levels or low magnesium levels are the two electrolyte deformities most linked to getting Torsades de pointes.

49. There are several types of heart block. Which type of heart block is considered to be the most severe?
    a. First degree heart block
    b. Second degree heart block Mobitz I
    c. Second degree heart block Mobitz II
    d. Third degree heart block

Answer: d. In third degree heart block, there is a dissociation between the atrial electrical impulse and the QRS (ventricular depolarization impulse). For this reason, the ventricular rate is very slow and the patient is generally very symptomatic.

50. What can be said about the atrial and ventricular rates in first degree heart block?
    a. The ventricular rate is independent of the atrial rate.
    b. The atrial rate and ventricular rate are the same.
    c. The ventricular rate is close to the atrial rate but there are missed beats.
    d. The ventricular rate is half the atrial rate.

Answer: b. In first degree heart block, there is a prolonged PR interval but there are no missed beats, so the atrial rate and ventricular rate are the same.

51. Why is a Mobitz II AV block considered worse than a Mobitz I AV block?
    a. The Mobitz II AV block tends to have more skipped beats than a Mobitz I AV block.

b. The Mobitz II AV block is associated with more distal disease in the conduction system.

c. The Mobitz II AV block is more likely to degenerate into a third-degree heart block when compared to a Mobitz I AV block.

d. The Mobitz II AV block has a slower heart rate than a Mobitz I AV block.

Answer: c. The main reason why a Mobitz II AV block is considered worse than a Mobitz I AV block is that it degenerates into third-degree AV block to a greater degree and carries a worse prognosis.

52. The patient has a pulse, tachycardia, a narrow QRS complex but an irregular rhythm. What is the least likely cause of the rhythm as can be seen on the rhythm strip?
   a. Atrial flutter
   b. Wandering atrial pacemaker tachycardia
   c. Atrial fibrillation
   d. Supraventricular tachycardia

Answer: d. Any of the above will yield tachycardia and an irregular rhythm except for SVT, which has an extremely regular rhythm and needs to be treated differently than any of the other listed rhythms.

53. The patient is stable with a pulse but has a wide-complex QRS and a rhythm strip showing ventricular tachycardia. What drug should be tried first?
   a. Epinephrine
   b. Diltiazem
   c. Amiodarone
   d. Diltiazem

Answer: c. The medical treatment of choice for this condition is amiodarone, which is given at 150 mg over ten minutes and repeated for a total of 2.2 grams in twenty-four hours. The ultimate treatment to restore normal sinus rhythm (NSR) is synchronized cardioversion.

54. In treating a patient who has an obvious Torsades de pointes rhythm, what should you give the patient to correct the rhythm disturbance?
   a. IV diltiazem
   b. IV magnesium
   c. IV adenosine
   d. IV propranolol

Answer: b. The treatment of choice for Torsades de pointes is IV magnesium, given as a short-term bolus followed by an infusion.

55. What is the first medication to consider giving in bradycardia, once an IV has been established?
   a. Dopamine

b. Epinephrine

c. Atropine

d. Sodium bicarbonate

Answer: c. Atropine should be given every three to five minutes for up to six doses before trying any other medication.

56. At what point does the patient require oxygen by nasal cannula or mask, even if they are not dyspneic?
    a. At any O2 sat if tachycardic
    b. At O2 sat levels of less than 97 percent
    c. At O2 sat levels of less than 95 percent
    d. At O2 sat levels of less than 94 percent

Answer: d. O2 sat levels of less than 94 percent should be treated with supplemental oxygen, even if the patient has no symptoms.

57. What is the treatment of choice for an unstable tachycardic rhythm of any etiology?
    a. Propranolol
    b. Synchronized cardioversion
    c. Diltiazem
    d. Digoxin IV

Answer: b. The treatment of choice for unstable tachycardia of any origin is to perform synchronized cardioversion with sedation, if possible.

58. The patient is in shock and shows signs of pulmonary edema. What is not considered an underlying etiology?
    a. Pump failure
    b. Volume depletion
    c. Abnormal heart rate (too fast or too slow)
    d. Pulmonary hypertension

Answer: d. Any of the above problems can account for pulmonary edema and shock except for pulmonary hypertension.

59. The patient is in shock without evidence for pulmonary edema and the etiology is unknown. What is the first treatment of choice once an IV has been established?
    a. Give a fluid bolus with crystalloid solution
    b. Give at least two blood transfusions
    c. Give IV albumin
    d. Give norepinephrine IV

Answer: a. The treatment of choice as a first-line agent for shock unassociated with pulmonary edema is to give a fluid bolus as a loss of fluid might be the cause of the problem or fluids may bring up the blood pressure.

60. The patient has pulmonary edema and an elevated blood pressure. What drug should be considered as a first-line agent?
    a. Dobutamine
    b. Nitroglycerin
    c. Dopamine
    d. Norepinephrine

Answer: b. With a normal blood pressure and pulmonary edema, the patient can have IV nitroglycerin, which will improve the pulmonary edema and decrease the blood pressure.

61. The patient has pulmonary edema and evidence of hypotension. The cause is unknown but the heart rate is normal. What is a first-line treatment if the patient has evidence of clinical shock?
    a. Norepinephrine
    b. Dobutamine
    c. Nitroglycerine
    d. Nitroprusside

Answer: a. The treatment of choice for pulmonary edema and shock is to start IV norepinephrine, which will restore perfusion and improve the blood pressure.

62. What is the recommended dose of amiodarone for ventricular fibrillation?
    a. 1 mg/min IV over ten minutes
    b. 300 mg IV push
    c. 150 mg IV push
    d. 0.5 mg/min infusion

Answer: b. When used for ventricular fibrillation, the recommended dose of amiodarone is 300 mg given intravenously as an IV push.

63. What is the maximum recommended dose of atropine in a cardiac arrest situation?
    a. One milligram
    b. Two milligrams
    c. Three milligrams
    d. Four milligrams

Answer: c. The maximum recommended dose of atropine is three milligrams total, given in doses of 0.5 to 1 mg at a time every three to five minutes.

64. What is a major contraindication to giving dopamine?
    a. Hypotension

b. Bradycardia

c. Shock

d. Hypovolemia

Answer: d. A major contraindication to giving dopamine is hypovolemia. The patient needs to be euvolemic before the drug can be used.

65. For which emergency situation is lidocaine not a recommended agent?
    a. Ventricular tachycardia
    b. Ventricular fibrillation
    c. Torsades de pointes
    d. Second degree heart block Mobitz II

Answer: d. Lidocaine is recommended in all of the above situations, except for second-degree AV heart block Mobitz II.

66. What is the maximum recommended dose of lidocaine when given in the treatment of ventricular tachycardia?
    a. 1 mg/kg
    b. 2 mg/kg
    c. 3 mg/kg
    d. 4 mg/kg

Answer: c. The maximum recommended dose of lidocaine in the management of ventricular tachycardia is 3 mg/kg.

67. For what arrhythmia is magnesium the first-line agent?
    a. Torsades de pointes
    b. Atrial flutter
    c. Second degree AV block Mobitz II
    d. Symptomatic bradycardia

Answer: a. The first-line agent for Torsades de pointes is magnesium, given intravenously.

68. What is the initial dose of procainamide in a cardiac arrest/ventricular tachycardia situation?
    a. 15-17 mg/kg IV over thirty minutes
    b. 15-17 mg/kg IV push
    c. 15-17 mg IV over one hour
    d. 15-17 grams IV over thirty minutes

Answer: a. The dose is about 15-17 mg/kg IV over thirty minutes up to a maximum dose of 1.5 grams. The infusion should be stopped if there is hypotension or prolongation of the QRS complex by 50 percent of the original length.

69. What is the main indication for bretylium in an ACLS situation?

112

a. Ventricular fibrillation

b. Supraventricular tachycardia

c. Hypertension

d. Torsades de pointes

Answer: a. The main indication for the use of bretylium in an ACLS situation is ventricular fibrillation that is unresponsive to the use of lidocaine and epinephrine. It is an antihypertensive but is not used in an ACLS situation where hypertension is the problem.

70. What is the initial dose of bretylium in an ACLS situation?

a. 1 mg per kg IV push

b. 5 mg per kg IV push

c. 10 mg per kg IV push

d. 15 mg per kg IV push

Answer: b. The initial dose of bretylium in an ACLS situation is five mg per kg IV push, followed by a 20-cc flush of fluids to allow the bretylium to circulate throughout the circulation.

71. What is the main indication for verapamil?

a. Ventricular tachycardia

b. Wide complex polymorphic tachycardia

c. Wolff-Parkinson-White syndrome with atrial fibrillation

d. Paroxysmal supraventricular tachycardia

Answer: d. The main use of verapamil is in the management of PSVT, for which it is a second-line agent.

72. What drug is successful in controlling the heart rate in atrial flutter when given as an infusion?

a. Verapamil

b. Diltiazem

c. Epinephrine

d. Atropine

Answer: b. Diltiazem is given as an infusion to control the heart rate in atrial flutter, given titrated intravenously and titrated to the heart rate.

73. What is the most common complication of hypoxia and under-ventilation in children?

a. Supraventricular tachycardia

b. Bradycardia

c. Sinus tachycardia

d. Frequent PVCs

Answer: b. The most common complication of hypoxia and under-ventilation in children is bradycardia, which will degenerate into asystole if not treated.

74. What is an option for giving drugs like epinephrine in a child with cardiac arrest?
    a. Interosseous bolus
    b. Intravenous bolus
    c. Intratracheal installation
    d. All of the above

Answer: d. Children may have problems with IV access but it is available for most children. Epinephrine can also be given by means of interosseous bolus or intratracheal instillation.

75. Which vital sign is out of the normal range for a toddler?
    a. Temperature of 98.6 degrees Fahrenheit
    b. Heart rate of 180 bpm
    c. Respiratory rate of 25 respirations per minute
    d. Blood pressure of 90/50

Answer: b. The vital signs are all normal except for the heart rate, which has an upper normal limit of 140 bpm in toddlers.

76. When the AED is ready and reads a shockable rhythm, what is the first shock intensity that should be delivered?
    a. Two joules per kilogram
    b. Four joules per kilogram
    c. Two joules
    d. Four joules

Answer: a. The first shock should be two joules per kilogram so an assessment of the weight of the child should be undertaken as soon as possible during an arrest situation.

77. Epinephrine is part of the pediatric cardiac arrest algorithm. What is the correct dose and timing of giving epinephrine to kids?
    a. 0.1 mg every three to five minutes
    b. 0.1 mg/kg every three to five minutes
    c. 0.1 mg/kg given once after the second shock
    d. 0.1 mg/kg given every ten minutes

Answer: b. The correct dosing of epinephrine in an arrest situation is 0.1 mg/kg every three minutes, given through intraosseous, intratracheal, or intravenous methods.

78. After epinephrine has been given and shocks have been delivered up to three times, what is a good next choice of treatment in a pediatric cardiac arrest?
    a. Lidocaine IV
    b. Procainamide IV
    c. Bretylium IV
    d. Sodium bicarbonate IV

Answer: a. Lidocaine at 5 mg/kg should be given as single IV dose after the third shock has failed to restore the child's cardiorespiratory status.

79. In sizing up the scene, what is the first consideration for the safety and care of everyone?
    a. Body substance precautions
    b. Scene safety
    c. Mechanism of injury assessment
    d. Triage the patients

Answer: a. Body substance precautions should be the first thing to consider. This may involve only having to put gloves on or get out an Ambu bag to ventilate the patient rather than doing mouth-to-mouth resuscitation.

80. Upon first assessing the patient, what is the first thing to assess?
    a. Airway
    b. Circulation
    c. Level of consciousness
    d. Breath rate

Answer: c. The level of consciousness should be quickly evaluated first and then the ABCs of airway, breathing, and circulation.

81. Where should the pulse be assessed in children or an infant?
    a. Radial artery
    b. Carotid artery
    c. Femoral artery
    d. Brachial artery

Answer: d. The brachial artery is the best place to check the pulse in an infant or child who is a victim of trauma.

82. What is the best way to assess the patency of the trauma patient's airway?
    a. Explore the mouth and throat with a flashlight.
    b. Talk to the patient and see if they talk normally back to you.
    c. Listen for breath sounds using a stethoscope.
    d. Get an oxygen saturation level.

Answer: b. The fastest and best way to evaluate the patency of the trauma patient's airway is to talk to the patient and see what kind of response you get. If the patient can talk normally, they likely have a patent airway.

83. What is the fastest way to assess whether or not oxygenation/ventilation is adequate?
    a. Get an oxygen saturation level
    b. Check the capillary refill

c. Count the respiratory rate

d. Get an arterial blood gas measurement

Answer: a. An oxygen saturation level is perhaps the best way to assess the oxygenation/ventilation adequacy of the patient. Arterial blood gases take too long and the respiratory rate alone does not say much about the adequacy of oxygenation. The capillary refill is a measurement of the adequacy of the circulation.

84. Under what condition might an ET tube not be indicated?
    a. An unconscious patient
    b. A patient with thoracic trauma
    c. A patient with head and neck trauma
    d. A patient with abdominal trauma

Answer: d. All of the above reasons are considered reasons why a person might be indicated to have an ET tube except for abdominal trauma, which by itself does not provide an indication for intubation.

85. What might be some signs of under-ventilation?
    a. Obtundation
    b. Belligerence
    c. Multiple rib fractures
    d. Any of the above

Answer: d. Things like obtundation, agitation, belligerence, multiple rib fractures, shallow breathing, and noisy breathing are all indicative of under-ventilation requiring further evaluation of the patient's oxygen level.

86. Why should an oropharyngeal airway be reserved for unconscious patients?
    a. Conscious patients usually have an intact airway.
    b. Conscious patients may vomit and aspirate with this airway.
    c. Conscious patients may not be able to talk with this airway.
    d. Conscious patients rarely need any ventilatory support.

Answer: b. The main reason why an oropharyngeal airway should be inserted only in unconscious patients is that conscious patients will gag on this airway, vomit, and possibly aspirate gastric contents.

87. What is the major contraindication for doing a nasopharyngeal airway in a trauma patient?
    a. Having a cribriform plate fracture suspected.
    b. Suspected of having a broken nose.
    c. Oropharyngeal bleeding.
    d. Semi-conscious patient.

Answer: a. Anyone suspected of having a cribriform plate fracture should not have a nasopharyngeal airway placed as it can travel up the broken plate and get into the brain tissue.

88. Which of the following drugs are used in rapid sequence intubation that will paralyze the patient for the procedure?
    a. Succinylcholine
    b. Etomidate
    c. Propofol
    d. Fentanyl

Answer: a. Of the above choices, only succinylcholine is a true muscle relaxant, which can be given prior to intubating the patient who isn't completely unconscious. It effectively paralyzes the patient.

89. What is the most common cause of shock in the trauma patient?
    a. Dehydration
    b. Sepsis
    c. Blood loss
    d. Cardiac pump failure

Answer: c. The main cause of shock in the trauma patient, particularly in the initial stages, is blood loss causing hypovolemia and lack of perfusion of the end organs.

90. What is a major cause of obstructive shock?
    a. Hypovolemia
    b. Cardiac tamponade
    c. Cervical spinal cord injury
    d. Severe head injury

Answer: b. Both a tension pneumothorax and cardiac tamponade can cause obstructive shock with a lack of ability of the heart to effectively pump blood around the body, resulting in hypotension and shock.

91. Which area of the body does not undergo vasoconstriction as an initial response to shock in a trauma patient?
    a. Viscera
    b. Skin
    c. Muscle
    d. Brain

Answer: d. There is vasoconstriction of the blood vessels leading to the stomach, skin, and viscera in order to preserve blood flow to the kidneys, heart, and brain.

92. What is considered the earliest sign of shock in a trauma patient?
    a. Tachycardia

b. Tachypnea

c. Decreased systolic blood pressure

d. Decreased pulse pressure

Answer: a. The first sign of shock in a trauma patient is compensatory tachycardia as the heart tries to increase the cardiac output by increasing the heart rate.

93. What is the most common cause of injuries in school-age children and teens?
   a. Bicycle injuries
   b. Suicide
   c. Homicide
   d. Motor vehicle accidents

Answer: a. Bicycle injuries account for the most injuries seen in school-age children and teens.

94. Among pediatric burn injury, what is the most common age group to sustain these types of injuries?
   a. 0-1 years
   b. 1-4 years
   c. 4-9 years
   d. 10-15 years

Answer: b. Pediatric burns tend to be seen in children aged one to four years of age. The other ages represent age groups that have a lesser incidence of burns.

95. What type of injury is the most common cause of death secondary to an injury in children?
   a. Penetrating thoracic injury
   b. Blunt abdominopelvic injury
   c. Closed head injury
   d. Penetrating abdominal injury

Answer: c. Closed head injuries not only cause a great degree of disability in children but are the most common cause of injury-related deaths in children under the age of 18 years.

96. What is not considered an indication to do a head CT in a child under the age of 2 years who has sustained a head trauma?
   a. Loss of consciousness for more than one minute
   b. Focal neurologic findings
   c. Multiple episodes of vomiting
   d. Poor feeding

Answer: d. All of the above are good reasons to do a CT scan of the head in a child under the age of two years who has sustained a head injury except for poor feeding, which can post-date a head injury that won't show anything on CT scan of the head.

97. Why is it better to use a ventriculostomy catheter to measure the ICP in children versus the Camino monitor?
   a. It can be used on kids of all ages and the Camino monitor cannot do this.
   b. It is a more accurate measurement of the ICP when compared to the Camino monitor.
   c. It can both measure the ICP and drain the fluid off, which isn't true of the Camino monitor.
   d. It is less invasive than the Camino monitor.

Answer: c. The biggest advantage of the ventriculostomy catheter in measuring the ICP is that it is both therapeutic (can draw fluid off the ventricles) and can measure the ICP at the same time.

98. You are managing the care of a child with an increased intracranial pressure from a head injury. What treatment are you least likely to use for this?
   a. IV mannitol
   b. Hyperventilation
   c. Sedation
   d. ICP drainage

Answer: b. Hyperventilation isn't recommended for children with an increased ICP because it causes vasoconstriction that adversely affects the brain. The other choices are good treatments for children who have an increased ICP.

99. What organ is most likely to be injured in a blunt trauma injury to a child's abdomen?
   a. Spleen
   b. Liver
   c. Kidneys
   d. Viscera

Answer: a. The spleen is the most likely organ to be injured in a blunt trauma incident affecting a child's abdomen, followed by the liver and kidneys.

100.   For what reason is a CT scan of the abdomen better than a diagnostic peritoneal lavage evaluation?
   a. CT scanning is faster than a DPL evaluation
   b. CT scanning can better identify the source of the bleeding than can a diagnostic peritoneal lavage
   c. CT scanning is not invasive and a DPL examination is highly invasive
   d. CT scanning is not better than a DPL examination because it involves radiation exposure

Answer: b. CT scanning is preferred over a DPL evaluation because it can identify the source of the bleeding better than a DPL test, which is nonspecific as to the source of the bleeding if it is detected.

Made in the USA
Columbia, SC
21 January 2024

30747475R00070